D0787657

VOLUME IV

INTEGRATIVE
MANUAL THERAPY

FOR THE CONNECTIVE TISSUE SYSTEM

Myofascial Release:
The 3-Planar Fascial Fulcrum Approach

Sharon (Weiselfish) Giammatteo, Ph.D., P.T., I.M.T., C.
Jay B. Kain, Ph.D., P.T., A.T.C., I.M.T., C.
Edited by Thomas Giammatteo, D.C., P.T., I.M.T., C.

North Atlantic Books
Berkeley, California

Published by
North Atlantic Books
P.O. Box 12327
Berkeley, California 94712

The following are service marks of Sharon (Weiselfish) Giammatteo/DCR:

3-Planar Fascial Fulcrum Approach[SM]	Longitudinal Fiber Therapy (LFT)[SM]
De-Facilitated Fascial Release[SM]	Muscle Energy and 'Beyond' Technique[SM]
Dialogues in Contemporary Rehabilitation[SM]	Myofascial Mapping[SM]
Horizontal Fiber Release[SM]	Neurofascial Process[SM]
Horizontal Fiber Therapy (HFT)[SM]	Soft Tissue Myofascial Release[SM]
Integrated Diagnostics[SM]	Synchronizer[SM]
Integrative Manual Therapy[SM], IMT[SM]	Synergic Pattern Imprint[SM]
Integrated Systems Approach[SM]	Synergic Pattern Release[SM]
Ligament Fiber Therapy[SM]	Tendon Release Therapy[SM]

For further information regarding DCR products and seminars, please contact:
Dialogues in Contemporary Rehabilitation
800 Cottage Grove Road, Suite 211
Bloomfield, Connecticut 06002
860-243-5220
www.centerimt.com/dcrhealth@aol.com

Original IMT series design by Andrea DuFlon. Series revisions and book production by A/M Studios.
Drawings by Ayelet Giammatteo Weiselfish and Alanna Heaney.
Photographs by John Giammatteo; case study photos courtesy DCR.

Distributed to the book trade by Publishers Group West.
Printed in the United States of America.

Integrative Manual Therapy for the Connective Tissue System is sponsored by the Society for the Study of Native Arts and Sciences, a nonprofit educational corporation whose goals are to develop an educational and crosscultural perspective linking various scientific, social, and artistic fields; to nurture a holistic view of arts, sciences, humanities, and healing; and to publish and distribute literature on the relationship of mind, body, and nature.

Library of Congress Cataloging-in-Publication Data
Weiselfish-Giammatteo, Sharon.
   Integrative manual therapy for the connective tissue system : myofascial release /
by Sharon (Weiselfish) Giammatteo and Jay B. Kain ; edited by Thomas A. Giammatteo.
     p. ; cm.
Includes bibliographical references and index.
Summary: "Provides detailed descriptions of hands-on techniques, with pictures and photographs, for decreasing pain and tension in the myofascial tissues"—Provided by publisher.
ISBN 1-55643-469-3 (cloth)
1. Myofascial pain syndromes. 2. Manipulation (Therapeutics)
I. Kain, Jay B. II. Giammatteo, Thomas. III. Title.
[DNLM: 1. Connective Tissue Diseases—therapy. 2. Musculoskeletal Diseases—therapy.
3. Musculoskeletal Manipulations—methods. 4. Physical Therapy Techniques. 5. Wounds
and Injuries—therapy. WD 375 W427i 2005]
RC927.3.W45 2005
616.7'4—dc22
                                                2004030010

1 2 3 4 5 6 7 8 9 10 DATA 09 08 07 06 05

ACKNOWLEDGMENTS

The culmination of this effort is only possible thanks to many wonderful people. Leading all acknowledgments must be mine to my co-author, Sharon (Weiselfish) Giammatteo. For without her persistent support and organizational skills, this text would have never been completed.

To Ayelet G. Weiselfish, for all her expertise in drawing and artistic talents, as well as doing many of the small things that make a project like this so successful.

To Tom Giammatteo, for all his behind-the-scenes technical support and consumate professionalism.

To the staff of Regional Physical Therapy, my colleagues, for their collective expertise, constant support, and development of the ideals of IMT.

To Mark Schooley, for his priceless friendship, endless support, and eloquence of heart.

To my wife Debby, and our children Alex, Jenny, and Caroline, for their constant love, and the support of the things I love to do.

To Robert Bergquist, and the late Sherrod Shaw, for their inspiration, care, and support during my informative professional years.

To Lisa Caul, in appreciation for her typing skills, friendship, and support, for all those last minute edits, and taking care of business when I needed it the most.

Jay B. Kain

My acknowledgment and thanks go to those who supported this project:

To Jay Kain, my partner and co-author, who has supported my development of Integrative Manual Therapy for over twenty years.

To Tom Giammatteo, whose brilliance in all aspects of manual therapy, computer technology and diagnostics provided comprehensive support throughout the development of this book.

To Ayelet G. Weiselfish, my daughter, who is with me at the start through finish of this and every other project.

To my partners and colleagues at Regional Physical Therapy in Connecticut, where research is performed with a team approach.

To our patients, who appreciate the therapy which contributes to their healing.

To our students, who provide feedback regarding their patients who are healing from Integrative Manual Therapy.

Sharon (Weiselfish) Giammatteo

TABLE OF CONTENTS

A WORD FROM THE AUTHORS

The purpose of this text is to present an effective and efficient method for addressing physical dysfunction. There is no panacea for removing all problems from the human body, yet there are some techniques that are quite comprehensive offering almost universal application. Our Myofascial Release 3-Planar Fascial Fulcrum Approach involving indirect neuromusculoskeletalfascial augmentations is such a technique. Dr. (Weiselfish) Giammatteo first presented it in 1981, and since that time many professionals have contributed to its development and enhancement. Though primarily a method for improving joint motion and tissue flexibility, the effects of treatment are far reaching and induce improvement in a wide range of dysfunction.

The techniques presented here have been utilized for acute and chronic clients, suffering from pediatric, orthopedic, geriatric, sports medicine and, neurologic disorders. Our protocols address both acute and severe inflammatory problems. Difficult and complex pathologies such as burns and non-union fractures benefit significantly when the methods are applied properly. Edema and lymphatic congestion, both acute and chronic, improve. First aide for sports injuries and trauma attain exceptional results with the Soft Tissue Myofascial Release technique. Old scars, fibromyalgia, myofibrositis, venous congestion, joint and soft-tissue adhesions will change within a few treatment sessions.

This Myofascial Release approach is indirect, gentle, and will integrate well with other manual approaches and electrotherapy modalities. Every person is a soul-driven being who responds from moment to moment to environmental factors with sensations and perceptions that, in turn, affect every aspect of the body's growth and development. At the same time, emotional energies allow, influence, inhibit, and restore changes in anatomy and physiology. Our approach, therefore, is most effective when applied in combination with various other manual therapies, taking into account multiple anatomic, physiologic, and energetic factors. With our combined understanding of Body, Mind, and Soul, our approach can facilitate improved therapeutic outcomes and enhanced quality of life.

All persons, both clients, and facilitators, are invited to use the protocols for Mysofascial Release given in this book, in spite of the fact that much controversy revolves around the general application of manual therapy. We hope that the following will put some of these considerations to rest.

Whenever there are serious medical problems, including specifically pathophysiology with indeterminable prognosis and pharmaceutical intervention, the client should consider involving the medical professional who is supervising their long-term care in their Myofascial Release program. When there is a history of systemic disorders, degenerative disease with fatal prognosis (for example, cancer), real organ impairment (including renal failure, cirrhosis of the liver, congestive heat failure, late stages of emphysema, or other serious problems), such conventional medical involvement is also recommended.

Otherwise, there are few precautions and no real contraindications for this approach. All clients can attain increased soft tissue flexibility and improved joint mobility. All persons can gain improved metabolic transport and circulation. (Of course, until there is more empirical clinical research with the above-mentioned patient populations, caution is always recommended.) When the therapist wishes to use the 3-Planar Myofscial Release Approach with a patient suffering from a severe ailment, professional responsibility includes the observation and documentation of all signs and symptoms, and the tracking for evidence of degenerative dysfunction enhancement. It is often advisable to assemble a multi-disciplinary team of professionals appropriate to the specific situation. For instance, for the functional rehabilitation program of a neurologic patient, a team consisting of an appropriate combination of an occupational therapist, physical therapist, physiatrist, speech therapist, and a cognitive therapist is recommended. Whenever an orthopedic or internal medicine referral is attached, there is an issue of practitioner responsibility for improved functional outcome. But when the medical situation is not severe and a client simply wishes to improve their well-being, he or she can even receive this therapy from a non-licensed practitioner.

The final measure of success is that a client should display improved objective status after treatment. This, therefore, can serve as a guideline for treatment. When there are no objective signs indicating improved posture, joint movement, flexibility, strength, function in daily living activities, this indicates, perhaps, that this approach is not the most appropriate. Of course, subjective indications of improvement are important too. These include decrease in pain and paresthesia; better balance, coordination, and movement; and an enhanced sense of well-being.

The authors offer this book as a resource both for further research and for clinical practice. Bibliographical references are provided throughout to assists the reader's investigations. The research presented in Part Six is the first of its kind, comprising quantitative research on 400 joints with severe and chronic deformities. The evidence from the statistical analysis of the research results is unequivocal and demonstrates objectively that effective management of chronic joint and soft tissue dysfunction is possible with this approach. We are confident that practical management of body dysfunction with Myofascial Release, A 3-Planar Fascial Fulcrum Approach, will bring further positive clinical results which, in turn, will stimulate further research by academicians and scientists. We therefore anticipate that new information on connective tissue pathology and related fields will be forthcoming over the next few years.

Sharon (Weiselfish) Giammatteo, Ph.D., P.T., I.M.T., C.
Jay B. Kain, Ph.D., P.T., A.T.C., I.M.T., C.

FOR THE LEARNER

Physical concepts are free creations of the human mind and are not, however it may seem, uniquely determined by the external world.... In our endeavor to understand reality we are somewhat like a man trying to understand the mechanism of a closed watch.... He sees the face and the moving hands, even hears it ticking, but has no way of opening the case; if he is ingenious, he may form some picture of the mechanism which could be responsible for all things he observes, but he may never be quite sure, so his picture is the only one which could explain his observations.... He will never be able to compare his picture with the real mechanism and he cannot ever imagine the possibility of measuring such a comparison.

Albert Einstein

PART ONE

THE CONNECTIVE TISSUE SYSTEM

CHAPTER 1

THE GENESIS OF MANUAL THERAPY

An historical examination of the beginnings and progress of manual therapy techniques may offer the practitioner a clear view of the roots to this part of our professional past. Unfortunately, there is no single path back through time regarding the origins of the art and science of manual therapy. The evidence of ancient wall paintings indicates that some kind of manual treatment existed in prehistoric cultures prior to the advent of written texts. Cantu, Grodin, and Juhan, among others, have reviewed numerous scholarly texts regarding the history of the ideals and philosophy behind modern manual therapy.

As soon as writing appears, specific mention of manual therapy appears in it. In the ancient Chinese medical text, *The Yellow Emperor's Classic of Internal Medicine* from as early as 2550 B.C., we find high praise for touch and hands-on approaches to intervention in pathology (Schoitz, 1958). Some time later, at about 400 B.C., the Greek physicians Hippocrates and Asclepiades record descriptions of manipulation, massage, and traction, with "repositioning" being a key focus of treatment (Cantu and Grodin 1992; Schoitz 1958). Galen, another Greek physician and author of approximately sixteen medical texts, documented early neurological investigations and noted, among other findings, the differentiation of motor and sensory nerves and identified seven cranial nerves. He placed a great emphasis on the spine and on the "repositioning of outward dislocations" (Cantu and Grodin 1992). He was one of the first practitioners to treat paresthesia and extremity pain by addressing dislocations of the spine (Cantu and Grodin 1992). References to illustrious practitioners in the field of physical medicine dot the literature throughout recorded history, and no doubt there

have been untold myriads of practitioners whose work has npot made it into the history books. One person's work who did get noticed was the Persian philosopher, theologian, and physician, Avicenna (c. 1000 A.D.), whose medical summaries include references to manual medicine. His work reiterated Hippocrates' findings and further validated this Greek's approach to intervention (Cantu and Grodin 1992). In the early to mid 1300s a physician named Guy de Chauliac authored a text that remained a cornerstone for surgical approaches for approximately two centuries. De Chauliac describes various manual approaches that were apparently applied simultaneously with surgery (Schoitz 1958).

A review of literature through the 1600s would reveal other individuals who perpetuated the practice of manual therapy and bodywork. A group of individuals in England popularized "bone setting," a technique that focuses on the repositioning of small, out-of-place bones to facilitate healing. At the time, more traditional medical practitioners branded the practice quackery, as most bonesetters had little formal education. After years of persistent observation and experiment on the part of courageous and insightful practitioners, the benefits of this approach were finally acknowledged by the medical profession. Bone setting remained prevalent through the middle of the 1800s, and the term is still in use today (Cantu and Grodin 1992).

At the present time, bonesetting is usually associated with osteopathy, a medical fielded for which the foundation was laid in 1874 by Dr. Andrew Taylor Still. The principal tenet of Still's osteopathic philosophy was that structural balance is the source for a healthy body. Still felt that dislocated bones, especially of the spine, as well as stressed or strained soft tissues adversely affect the body's overall homeostasis (Cantu and Grodin 1992). These ideas appear to be a continuation of the ideas of the original bonesetters. Still hypothesized that structural balance is necessary for the human organism to tap into its self-corrective capabilities. Without this balance, mechanical stress and strain on neurovascular structures facilitate pathology. The present authors use the following adage, essentially derived from Still's hypothesis, as a basis for much of their practice: *Structure dictates function, while function influences structure.*

Osteopathy has gained recognition within the traditional medical hierarchy over the past decades, but not without some loss of identity. In the United States today, osteopaths share almost all of the same practice privileges as their allopathic colleagues, while in other countries they have been placed under far more regulations and restrictions. That is to say, in this country osteopaths have become virtually indistinguishable from conventional physicians. Many of the current graduates of osteopathic schools appear to be specializing in traditional allopathic approaches for care giving, i.e., pharmacological approaches. Still's ideas about the treatment of individual cases are far removed from today's "meat market" philosophy of health care, where dollars dictate services, symptoms localize pathology, and advancing technology rather than deepening skill is the state of the art in patient care!

Another profession searching for an identity within the general health care spectrum is Chiropractic. As osteopaths fill many of the traditional roles of the allopathic practitioners, the chiropractic physician is gaining broader acceptance in their professed specialty: manipulation of the spine and extremities. Chiropractic started in the late 1800s when David Palmer branched out from his osteopathic roots to develop his own philosophy of manual intervention. His discovery, which he claimed was a new science, appears to be a combination of osteopathic medicine and other ancient Hipprocratic methods (Cantu and Grodin 1992). Palmer chartered a philosophy, which was referred to as the "Law of the Nerve." There are five basic tenets to this philosophy: (1) *subluxation* of the *vertebrae;* (2) that this subluxation will affect the structures that pass through the intervertebral foramina inclusive of blood, nerves and lymph vessels; (3) that this causes a disruption of function anywhere along the nerve distribution of that segmental level; (4) that this disinnervation leads to dysfunction and susceptibility to disease; and (5) adjustment or repositioning of vertebrae will release tensions and return normal innervations to the dysfunctional organs or receptor sites.

Despite the constant insults from the allopathic profession, chiropractic has survived and even gained a noticeably respectable niche in the health-care realm. And, as the chiropractor moves up the hierarchical, health-care ladder, manual physical therapists appear poised to make similar advances.

Traditionally, the focus of manual therapy had been on restoration of structure and on reduction of pain in order to facilitate healing; but over time, the static structural approach to treatment was slowly replaced by the addition of mobility and selective tension tests. By the late 1800s and early 1900s proponents of manual medicine were becoming more precise in their evaluation procedures.

In 1920, Edgar Cyriax became one of the first modern practitioners to embrace a manual approach to treatment. His work was furthered by his son, James Cyriax, who wrote two landmark texts that are still widely read and respected today.

Dr. James Cyriax's way of performing differential diagnoses was based on specific selective tensions of soft tissues with ensuing treatment reflecting the findings of those assessments (Cyriax 1947/1977). A younger contemporary of James Cyriax's, James Mennell, focused his research and writings on the importance of *joint mechanics*. He introduced and integrated the concept of *accessory joint motion*. While James Cyriax was a fervent supporter of the discogenic origins of back pain, James Mennell demonstrated how the *synovial joints* are responsible for many back complaints. Mennell outlined specific etiologic factors that could cause such joint pains and introduced important terminology that has exceptional significance today. This terminology includes: (1) *"joint play,"* (2) *"joint dysfunction,"* and (3) *"joint manipulation."* Mennell provided evidence that the mobilization of tissues in a specific manner creates normal joint balance and restoration of movement. The importance of local tissue extensibility is vital to recapturing normal motion (Mennell 1945).

Another proponent of mobility was the Norwegian physical therapist Freddy Kaltenborn. He derived the convex/concave rule of joint and osseous motion. Kaltenborn accounted for movement at both the articular surface and the distal lever arm respectively. He expanded his understanding of both components (joints and soft tissue) as being part of a greater whole, and consequently developed the realm of manual technique. Many researchers, including those mentioned already, have added to the effectiveness and efficacy of manual therapy.

More recently, Stanley Paris addressed a common problem in the evaluation and treatment of pathology. Placing emphasis on treating the dysfunction and not the pain, he reasoned that there is a high correlation between dysfunction and pain. If one treated the dysfunction, the pain would in most cases be positively affected. He expanded his concepts by adding definitions for component and joint accessory motionsand by categorizing types of manipulation. He hypothesized that treated soft tissues would improve in extensibility and that manipulations would produce additional positive neurophysiological effects.

While Paris utilized distraction, oscillations, and thrust manipulations to change joint and soft

tissue, Geoffrey Maitland refined an oscillatory technique to produce similar results. He perfected a graded oscillation approach that also helped modulate pain by neurophysiological means. He described four levels of oscillation with at least one level having two parts.

Most of the research reviewed since the beginning of the twentieth century has dealt with treating localized tissues in a direct manner. In other words, if a mechanical barrier in a soft tissue or joint is encountered during some selective tissue tension exam, the practitioner uses some level of graded force to push through the restriction. Fred Mitchell Sr., an osteopath, has contributed a procedure called *Muscle Energy Technique* whereby a joint is taken through a restriction in a direct, graded manner. The patient initiates a muscle contraction just before the soft tissue barrier (interbarrier zone) that apparently helps facilitate a repositioning of the malaligned structure.

In contrast with these "direct" techniques, Lawrence Jones has developed a treatment that is classified as an "indirect." Instead of moving a body part directly *into* a barrier, tissues are mobilized in a direction of ease. The practitioner places the tissue in a shortened position instead of trying to lengthen it. Indirect techniques, as we shall see, play a major role in the Myofascial Release Approach discussed in this book.

One can see that manual therapy approaches have evolved from a repositioning of a structure and the modulation of pain to mobility assessment and trying to understand more about causalgia with less focus on pain symptomology.

Many modalities of treatment dveloped throughout the twenthieth century, and many more being developed so today, do not confine themselves to the joint and the immediate surrounding soft tissues. Several explorers have recognized the importance of treating tissues far removed from a soft tissue problem at a local joint. These treatments can sometimes extend beyond the *dermatomal, myotomal, enterotomal,* and *sclerotomal* boundaries. The techniques they employ are based upon what the authors hypothesize to be a *neuro-reflexogenic* reaction. In the 1970s, for instance, John Upledger noted global treatment effects through the treatment of the *craniosacral* mechanism. As early as 1981, Sharon (Weiselfish) Giammatteo called attention to the importance of accounting for structures beyond local joints and soft tissues. She approached somatic dysfunction from an integrated systems viewpoint. She addressed pathology by assessing how each system directly or indirectly affects the etiology and its correlation.

Focus on the body in its entirety seemed logical from these author's points-of-view. Connective tissue represents an ubiquitous structure, the manipulation of which can produce treatment reactions that extend beyond basic physiologic boundaries. Jean Pierre Barral's work and Frank Lowen's practical adaptation of it, as well as his own research, represent safe, non-invasive treatment approaches that place the fascial system at the core of many dysfunctions. Current state of the art approaches utilized by (Weiselfish) Giammatteo and Lowen take the body beyond the "systems" formula. The application of principles derived from quantum physics to manual techniques has added greater effectiveness and efficiency and has decreased stress on the patient and practitioner alike. An example of this application is illustrated in techniques that acknowledge that "joint spaces" need treatment and maintenance as often as articular interfaces. Lowen and (Weiselfish) Giammatteo view joint spaces all together as an integral entity responsible for multiple static and dynamic physiologic functions. They have expanded the concept of joint spaces to a macroscopic and clinical level and hypothesized that all joint spaces collectively comprise a functional network throughout the body.

CHAPTER 2

AN OVERVIEW OF FASCIAL MANIPULATION

The attempted manipulation of various connective tissue components has lead to the development of a variety of techniques and approaches whose focus has been "fascial" in nature. The following is a brief overview of several "fascial" approaches. Cantu and Grodin review some of the approaches succinctly (Cantu and Grodin 1958). We suggest referring to their text for a more in-depth summary of those techniques and approaches. We present here but a synopsis of their original contributions.

Cantu and Gordin discuss Bindgewebbs Massage, an autonomic/reflexive approach to fascial manipulation using connective tissue massage. First developed in the 1920s by a German physiotherapist, Elizabeth Dicke, the technique relies on reflex pathways mediated through the autonomic nervous system in order to facilitate a therapeutic effect. Bindgewebbs Massage is performed systemically. It is also performed systematically. It specifies the number of strokes, the side of body to work on first, and even which fingers the practitioner should use in giving treatment. Though the approach is considered a superficial technique, its effects and potential application should not be under-emphasized. Dicke's purely "mechanical" technique was one of the first to specifically outline the exact "how to's" of this kind of treatment.

In general, beyond the correct mechanical application of technique, the energy transference associated with touch and the importance of treatment components such as focus and intention need further examination. Our clinical research has repeatedly revealed that good results with fascial release *can* be attained when an individual performs a technique mechanically. This means that hand placement alone, for a certain amount of time, is enough for eliciting good outcome.

Better results are obtained, however, when therapists apply mental focus or intention to the treatment structures. These better results include observable changes in many systems. The lymphatic systems show decreased edema. The circulatory system exhibits arrhythmia and warmth. Muscle and fascia reveal increased ranges of motion. Improved posture occurs in the skeletal system, and the nervous system produces less pain. Also, associated metabolic changes occur when these systems are affected. In many circumstances, the impact of intention alone, when dealing with multiple energy patterns in a treatment area, can provide the difference between major treatment responses in multiple systems as opposed to merely minor regional responses localized to the affected area. Thus, reflex connections have the potential to extend well beyond the superficial fascial system. By reflexively decreasing aberrant stimuli through dermatome, myotome, scleratome, or enterotome, we can affect the afferent firing signal and ultimately the efferent firing signal of a facilitated segment.

Another modified technique that is classified as "reflexive" since it deals primarily with reflexes is Hoffa Massage. The technique requires that the force used be gentle and elicit as little pain as possible. Other truly reflexive and energetic approaches include Foot Reflexology, Auriculotherapy, Acupressure, Zero Balancing and Polarity Therapy. Many reflexive pathways are poorly understood by traditional physiology and are better explained by energetic concepts such as mechano-energetic concepts from the field of applied quantum physics.

When any manual therapy technique utilizes a subtle yet gentle approach, there appears to be some component of reflex reaction that facilitates the relaxation of tissues. This in turn allows for deeper access to other tissues or creates an altered metabolic environment in the regional tissues addressed. The clinical experience of authors from associated professions has found a light exact touch is far more powerful when dealing with global or local somatic dysfunction than a more direct and aggressive touch or contact. A lighter touch that allows the body "to speak" is far more efficacious in stimulating the natural corrective powers of these tissues. Many practitioners, therefore, use gentle light forces as keystones to their practice and art.

Barral notes in his visceral work that the inherent protective nature of the body is a constant in which any forceful manipulation of tissues will either, in the short term or in the long term, cause the patient harm. In other words, the short-term gains attained with forceful measures are eventually lost by the body's reactive protective nature. Barral notes that this is especially true with the manipulation of the small intestines and kidneys, both of which are extremely reactive to force. In response to forceful manipulation the kidneys have a tendency to fracture, and the small intestines tend to create adhesions.

Cantu and Grodin (Cantu and Grodin 1958) reviewed two fascial approaches considered by them mechanical in nature namely, Rolfing and Trager. Ida Rolf introduced Rolfing with the intent of improving the body's balance in relation to gravity. The treatment technique is not based on a patient's current physical status or symptomology but on a regimented, ten-session protocol that addresses the different body quadrants. Additionally, Rolf noted that the body and mind are inseparable and that both need addressing in an integral manner when treatment is undertaken.

Milton Trager developed a therapeutic approach focusing on the subconscious mind. His techniques combine passive motions including rotation and traction plus active motions termed "Mentastics." Trager felt that the combination of the relaxation of the tissue and neuromuscular

re-education creates a powerful tool to help change poor postural habits and dysfunction. Trager's approach employs movement as a mechanical tool and is therefore classified as a "movement" approach. Other fascial techniques deemed mechanical include Shiatsu, Myotherapy, and Chua Ka.

Another approach combining mechanical and movement aspects was introduced by Joseph Heller in 1970. His form of bodywork, termed "Hellerwork," was initiated after he had practiced Rolfing for years. Hellerwork focuses on the body's connective tissues, i.e., the fascia, in relation to gravity, just as in Rolfing. He attempted to decrease tension in the fascia through body realignment. He saw that the more vertical a person remains, the less overall energy is consumed bracing against the effects of gravity. The person, therefore, has energy to perform the other activities of daily living. Hellerwork incorporates movement re-education based on exercises that mimic everyday movement and that reinforce stress-free methods of performance. Another component of his work includes a dialoguing technique designed to help connect mental patterns to their somatic expression.

The patient assumes different roles with each of the aforementioned techniques. With Chua Ka, Myotherapy, Shiatsu, Hoffa, and general connective tissue massage the patient is passive. Some of the mechanical techniques are part passive and part active, as is the case with Rolfing, Trager, and Hellerwork. Movement approaches necessitate the patient's participation in the therapy. Under the guidance of a practitioner, movements and postures are utilized to modify and change erratic or dysfunctional patterns that compromise static and dynamic motion. Whereas modalities that use the reflexive, mechanical, and autonomic approaches exemplify the first part of the adage mentioned above: "structure dictates function." Movement approaches illustrate how "function influences structure." In this case, the "structure" is the connective tissue. Four popular, exclusively movement approaches are: Alexander Techniques, Feldenkrais Technique, Aston Patterning, and Functional Orthopedics.

Alexander Technique relies on the functional position of the head and neck in relation to the rest of the body. The head and neck act as a primary control mechanism around which all else is coordinated. F.M. Alexander saw the head and neck as not only being representative of dysfunctional patterns elsewhere in the body, but also as the key to their correction. He found that if he superimposed normal movement patterns, poor postural habits would be eliminated. His work was supplemented by mechanical approaches that prepared a person for movement re-education.

Moshe Feldenkrais published his classic text, *Awareness Through Movement,* in 1971. He based his work on the treatment of dysfunctional movement patterns. He considered all persons as being essentially disabled in one manner or another. This is typified by his two-fold approach to treatment. First he focused on changing old habits and patterns that existed secondary to trauma; then he utilized a hands-on approach to slowly change inadequate movement into efficient movement. As with Alexander Technique, all new patterns are learned.

Alexander and Feldenkreis discovered an important aspect of learning new movement patterns. They realized that new learning is mediated through the cerebrum and eventually transferred to the cerebellum. They were aware that permanent postural changes are better achieved if the pattern is not the result of conscious behavior. When new learning is processed on a cerebral level only, the newly learned activities are quite often forgotten by the client. For this reason, many postural exercise programs meet with failure. Posture is reflexive in nature, not cerebral. The functional aspects of both of these programs, as well as Judith Aston's, appear to take this fact into account.

Judith Aston introduced her Aston Patterning in 1977. It is based on the concept that each body maintains and expresses patterns which can help or hurt the individual (Aston 1993). A person's mental and physical history can be expressed through the body. By learning how to evaluate a person three dimensionally, a practitioner can identify areas of stress and tension in the body's connective tissues. The practitioner facilitates an individual's journey in negotiating a balance of the body's tissue through touching, sensing and hearing.

Another method, Functional Orthopedics, introduced by Greg Johnson, combines mechanical techniques and movement pattern similar to the above mentioned practitioners. His movement patterns include stabilization, proprioceptive neuromuscular facilitation constructs, as well as direct connective tissue manipulation.

CHAPTER 3

PALPATION

Palpatory skills are essential for intermediate and advanced levels of myofascial work. Introductory and beginning levels of myofascial release require essentially very limited perceptive capabilities. Good to very good outcomes can be achieve almost mechanically. The most basic palpatory skill is that of "fascial glide." Using a light, moderate, or heavy contact, the practitioner compares fascial/soft tissue mobility in all three cardinal planes: sagittal, coronal and transverse. The practitioner must be familiar with all regional tissue anchors, visceral concerns, spinal relationships, rib/sternum/clavicle involvements, pelvic, sacral and coccyx inter-relationships, as well as weight-bearing versus non-weight-bearing considerations of soft and hard tissues. With practice, these and other basic constructs of fascial release can be performed mechanically in a competent manner. Unfortunately, there are many considerations regarding tissue and movement that directly and indirectly affect the integrated balance of the body beyond basic fascial release technique and that are beyond the reach of basic myofascial release techniques.

A significant component of intermediate and advanced myofascial technique deals with the practitioner's perception. Reliable perceptive capabilities allow a practitioner to focus on tissues locally and globally at the same time, as well as assess the depth of the problem. In other words, a three dimensional proximal picture can be examined and, at the same time, all of the rest of the body's influence can be factored in to give a complete appraisal of the problem. All physical diagnoses, performed manually, require a nearly instantaneous recognition of local and distal fascial/soft tissue strain patterns. Beyond this there are other factors present within the body that the

practitioner must be cognizant of. Such factors would include the ever-changing level of pressures within the different cavities of the body. The manual practitioner needs to understand how this system of pressures relates to our static and dynamic equilibrium so that palpatory findings can be interpreted accurately.

The manual practitioner should also be able to recognize the many inherent body rhythms such as the cranial, fascial, visceral, osseous, neural, and cardiac rhythms, to name but a few. It becomes clear that discerning the different layers of the muscle fiber i.e., *endomysium, perimysium,* and *epimysium,* is important, but less so when the vascular flow and neural input are integrated into the picture.

Finally, the skilled practitioner should be able to discern the depth of isolated problems as well as discriminate between structural and tissue boundaries at those levels. Palpation and differentiation between minute structures such as the layers of a muscle, nerve, or vascular structure are possible for the trained hand. In addition to these abilities, the authors have noted in relation to thousands of patients that the more focused a practitioner is in regards to a target structure, the faster the treatment results and the greater its effectiveness. In other words, the more a practitioner can account for multiple components, including perceptions of the depth, texture, density, temperature, quality, size, shape, contour, and mobility of tissues, the greater the treatment outcomes.

Accurate assessment of normal versus abnormal variations in regional internal pressure is also important for treatment outcomes. For example, palpatory perception of sub-atmospheric pressures in the thoracic cavity is different from the pressure gradients witnessed in the abdomen and cranium. Understanding sub-atmospheric pressure in the thorax and its influences on the rest of the body is essential in setting clinical expectations. Assessment of these inherent pressures can help modify treatment protocols and procedures.

The recognition of body rhythms helps the advanced practitioner to achieve truly integrated results within and among all the systems, including the energetic processes. The acknowledgement of individual body tissue rhythms and motilities has opened many opportunities for treatment outcome protocols. Since the beginning of the 1990s, accessing multiple body rhythms has accelerated our treatment expectations even with the most difficult systems pathologies. Arteries, veins, lymph, the lobes of the brain, and chambers of the heart have distinct and palpable rhythms. Organ rhythms, called "motilities," occur within both the fascial envelopes and the individual *parenchymal cells*. There are combination rhythms for structure as well. Each lobe of the brain and the brain stem has an individual motility, but the brain has an individual motility representative of all the lobe motilities combined. This rhythm is located at the *insula*. Certain organs have motilities reciprocal with each other, but some also have symmetrical motilities as well. There are also vital visceral and intervisceral movements and rhythms.

In addition to these organ rhythms, every structural unit in the body has a rhythm. The craniosacral rhythmic impulse is but one important rhythm, the discovery of which has helped advance the understanding of the interconnectedness of the body. The skeletal system, once thought to be inert, has been found to have multiple rhythms on multiple planes.

New applications of palpatory skills will assuredly yield more and different body rhythms in the future. Their importance cannot be overstated. The more we accept the common sense approach to these complex signals offered by the body (the fact that it makes sense that they should be there), the more we'll be able to unlock additional secrets to otherwise ubiquitous pathologies.

In our clinics we have also found consistent, reproducible dysfunction rhythms throughout the body indicative of many types of "medical model" dysfunction, including membrane dysfunction and infection motilities. Dysfunctional patterns are indicative of systemic or local problems. This has been investigated and tested for less than two years at the time of this writing (January, 2004) and will be being looked into clinically for some time to come.

Another constraint upon proper palpation is the fact that in order to palpate accurately it is necessary to be able to locate local restrictions along global lines of tension throughout the body. These lines, when deciphered, offer fast and easy ways to treat the keystone or core problem in any given situation. This is at the core of several "listening" techniques including Lowen's, Chauffour's, (Weiselfish) Giammatteo's, and Barral's.

Additionally, it must be understood that restriction and dysfunction rarely stand alone. It's probably safe to say that no dysfunction is truly independent. An area of restriction is restriced both in the sense of being restricted within a given system and as involving restrictions in other systems to which it might be in some way connected.

These applications of palpation skills raise the level of expectation of the practitioner and allow him/her to get close to the core issues of pathology and dysfunction. They are skills that should become an art for all manual therapists.

CHAPTER 4

CONNECTIVE TISSUE STRUCTURE AND FUNCTION

Understanding the concept of fascial release begins with a familiarity with the basic components of connective tissue. These tissues can be somewhat arbitrarily divided into two basic elements: cells and the extra-cellular matrix. This distinction underlies the complexity of the functional mix. Tissues comprise the matrix of the body and are composed of cellular elements, their precursors, and their derivatives. Cell ratios vary widely among different types of connective tissue, as does the make up of the extra-cellular matrix, i.e., protein fibers and ground substance.

From a holistic point of view, the body has four basic kinds of tissue: (1) epithelial tissue for protection, secretion, and absorption; (2) muscle tissue for contraction; (3) nerve tissue for sensation and conductivity; and (4) connective tissue for support, nutrition, defense, coordination, separation, balance, movement, and shock absorption. From the point of view of technical observation, connective tissue as a whole can be considered as an organ or as a single system. The connective tissue system includes all of the components derived from the mesenchyme, i.e., the *embryologic mesoderm*. These include: *ground substance, elastin, collagen, reticulin, bone, adipose, cartilage, pericardium, joint capsules, ligaments, tendons, nerve sheaths, muscle sheaths, blood and blood vessel walls, lymph and lymph vessels,* and *aponeuroses.* The connective tissue forms a continuous, contiguous system throughout the expanse of our body. Without the supportive framework of this system, one would be left with a mass of limp epithelial tissue, vacillating muscle, and nerve cells with no practical ability to function. Connective tissues comprise approximately 16 percent of our total body weight and store 23 percent of the body's total water content. In essence, connect tissue represents the glue that holds us together or keeps us from coming apart, depending on which viewpoint you prefer.

A close look at connective tissue and its components is warranted for the manual therapist: the great extent of this system can be appreciated by an examination of its pertinent parts. As mentioned in the introduction, the therapist who touches a patient with a positive intent will always have some therapeutic effect on the individual. This effect is mediated through multiple tissues and their derivatives. Essentially, any manual approach to treatment results in some form of fascial release.

As one of the body's basic tissues, connective tissue is actually subdivided into *connective tissue proper,* bone and cartilage, and blood and lymph. Connective tissue proper is further subdivided into *loose irregular (areolar), dense (fibrous),* and *regular* and *irregular connective tissues.* (See Table I.)

In general, connective tissue function is well known for its biomechanical as well as for its physiologic and metabolic roles. Connective tissues are involved directly and indirectly in every system in the body. They not only have intra-system connections, but also inter-system relationships. The synchronization of motion between all types of joints is directly related to the biochemical, intrasystem properties of connective tissue. This includes hard joints (bone on bone, including *fibro-* and *hyaline-cartilage articulations* in the body); soft joint (muscle to muscle, muscle to ligament, ligament to tendon, *bursa* to tendon, organ to organ); and partial soft joints (tendon to *tuberosity,* muscle to bone, organ to bone).

Loose connective tissue provides a pathway

for the *reticuloendothelial system* to interact with blood, lymph, and organs in order to fight infection. This is an example of an inter-system relationship. Connective tissues, therefore, mechanically act to provide a structural framework for protection, support, locomotion, coordination, and shock absorption for the body. These tissues differentiate into many forms to yield this function. They include bone, fascia, tendon, cartilage, ligaments, and other tissue. The metabolic and physiologic functions of connective tissues include protection from foreign pathogens, infection, and inflammation; transporting and storing vital nutrients for other tissues; eliminating waste products and toxins; and providing an avenue of communication between and among various tissues. The connective tissues defined here include blood, lymph, and loose connective tissue. In essence, the connective tissues represent the one system that connects all the other systems. It has been noted that connective tissue is so encompassing that components of every cell in the body have a relationship with it, and that were all other formal systems to dissolve and leave only the connective tissues, each of us would easily be recognizable; we would still retain enough finite features to be identified by sight!

Table I
Connective Tissue Differentiation (Three Major Classifications)

Connective Tissue Proper

Loose Connective Tissue differentiates into:

1. Areolar Connective Tissue
2. Adipose Tissue
3. Reticular Tissue

Dense Connective Tissue differentiates into:

1. Dense Regular Connective Tissue
   a. Tendons
   b. Ligaments
   c. Aponeuroses
   d. Fascia
   e. Elastic Tissue
2. Dense Irregular Connective Tissue
   a. Capsule
   b. Skin

Ground substance of connective tissue proper: Syrupy sticky consistency. Proteoglycans made up of glycoproteins and glycosaminoglycans attached to hyaluronic acid.

Fluid Connective Tissue

Blood differentiates into:

1. Red blood cells (erythrocytes)
2. White blood cells (leukocytes)

Lymph: Lymphocytes

Ground substance of fluid connective tissue: Plasma, more watery and fluid than ground substance of connective tissue proper.

Supportive Connective Tissue

Cartilage differentiates into:

1. Hyaline Cartilage
2. Fibro-Cartilage
3. Elasto-Cartilage

Bone

Ground Substance of supportive connective tissue: Referred to as the Matrix. Can range from a firm gel in cartilage to a solid matrix in bone secondary to the combinations of calcium, salts, and collagen fibers.

CHAPTER 5

THE CELLULAR COMPONENTS OF CONNECTIVE TISSUE

The cellular makeup of connective tissue varies markedly from tissue to tissue as do the fibrous component ratios and ground substance consistency. All connective tissues have these three components: cells, fiber, and ground substance. The *fibroblast* is the primary secretory cell for all three components. The fibroblast synthesizes all the major fibrillar components of connective tissue, including *collagen, elastin,* and *reticulin.* It also synthesizes the ground substance. As the fibroblast matures, it transforms and becomes the most prominent cellular element in normal connective tissue. Once mature, no further differentiation is noted in regard to component synthesis. The fibroblast becomes a *fibrocyte.* We will discuss the fibroblast further when we present our discussion of collagen production (see "The Origin of Collagen: Fibrillogenesis" in Chapter 6).

Undifferentiated cells in adult connective tissues retain the ability to transform into other specialized cells, depending on local needs. Not only can these cells transform, they can multiply. For example, a *macrophage* exists as a large round shaped cell called a *monocyte,* with no apparent specialized function until there is some pathological condition. Once that condition arises, the monocyte migrates to the involved area, transforms into a macrophage, and presents a front line defense as a *phagocytizing cell.* Macrophages are classified as either "fixed" or "free." Some of the fixed macrophages have the ability, when stimulated, to detach and act as "free" or "wandering" macrophages. The macrophages are scattered through the connective tissues. Once stimulated by the immune system they migrate towards a damaged area. This process is called *chemotaxis.* Stimulation occurs from chemicals released by damaged tissue or pathogens. Due to *endothelial*

system (immune system) stimulation, their numbers increase as well as their activity. Once a monocyte enters a damaged area or passes through the marginalized area of endothelial cells via the process called *diapedesis,* it changes to a macrophage and begins phagocytizing material. A single macrophage can ingest up to one hundred bacteria as well as neurotoxic material before it itself is phagocytized. It also has the ability to join other macrophages to help ingest extra large particles of debris. These are referred to as *giant phagocytic cells.* The macrophages are identified by regional location and have been given different names such as *histiocytes* (found in subcutaneous tissue and skin), *Langerhans cells* (found in epithelia and the digestive tract), and *microglia* (found in the central nervous system). Although there are many regional names, these specialized cells are all still macrophages. (See Table II.)

Another component of connective tissue is the *mast cells.* These are large cells found mainly near blood vessels. (See Figure 1.)

Mast cells have a dual function: (1) to secrete *histamine* (for *vasodilatation*); and (2) to secrete *heparin* (to prevent clotting). Additionally, these cells have been found to secrete *serotonin* and *bradykinin* during inflammatory situations. They also work closely with *basophils* during allergic reactions. Mast cells have been considered responsible for the production of some of the ground substance. This is based on staining results and the appearance of large numbers of these cells concentrated in regions undergoing healing. Mast cells have been postulated as an *end organ mediator* in the relationship between *ACTH* and *cortisone,* and are also associated with precancerous states in the skin.

Still another important component of connective tissue is the *plasma cells*. These cells, like other components, are found in infectious conditions. (See Figure1.) They produce antibodies in reaction to infectious states of connective tissue. Plasma cells develop from *lymphocytes*. Along with *microphages* (special phagocyte cells of the blood, i.e., *esinophils* and *neutrophils*), they relate directly to tissue damage and repair. The plasma cells are also responsible for *antibody* production. The lymphocytes, precursors of the plasma cells, are derived from the bone marrow in small supply, yet come mostly from *lymphoid tissues*. These cells attach themselves to their prey and act as a phagocytizing element, as do the macrophages. The lymphocyte can make many trips through the blood/lymph cycle, as its life span is around 100 to 300 days.

Another group of cells that reacts as part of our *reticuloendothelial system* and are found in the connective tissues, is the *granulocytes* or *polymophisms*. These names are derived from the way they look under a microscope. They are specialized cells including neutrophils, basophils, and esinophils. These three granulocytes plus the monocytes, lymphocytes, and plasma cells constitute the generally accepted subclassifications of white blood cells or *leukocytes*. Neutrophils comprise 62 percent of the white blood cell count. Together with the monocytes, neutrophils constitute our strongest front line defense against foreign bodies. They can phagocytize anywhere from 5 to 25 bacteria before they are absorbed. These components (monocytes and granulocytes) are derived from the bone marrow.

There is one more type of cell to be considered: a derivative of the *hemocytoblast* and

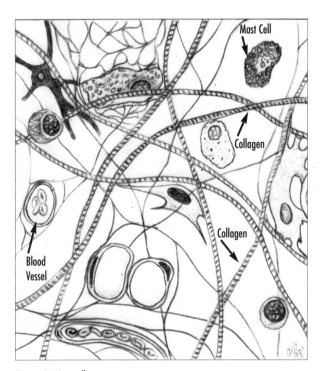

Figure 1. Mast cell.

myeloid stem cell differentiation. The myeloid stem cell transforms into a *megokaryocyte,* and the fragmentation of this huge cell leads to the formation of *platelets*. These cells, again, are active daily for damage control. They activate the blood clotting mechanism.

Lastly, there are other cells that are fixed to the connective tissues and have lesser or greater roles depending on regional needs. These include *melanocytes, adipocytes,* and mesenchymal cells. (See Table II and Figure 1.) Outside of the cellular milieu of connective tissue, there are fibrillar components that constitute an important part of the whole extramatrix picture.

Table II

Histological Make-Up of the Connective Tissue: Cellular Components

1. **Fibroblasts:** Fixed stellate shaped cells that produce all the fibrous components of connective tissue proper as well as the ground substance.

2. **Macrophages:** First line of defense for tissues against infection, inflammation, trauma, burns, etc.
   a. **Fixed Macrophages:** These are scattered throughout the connective tissues, and, when stimulated, can mobilize themselves and become free macrophages.
   b. **Free Macrophages:** Highly mobile versions of fixed macrophages but performing apparently the same functions.
   - Macrophages are named according to the tissues they are present in:
     1. Kuppfer cells in liver;
     2. Tissue macrophages in spleen, lymph, and bone marrow;
     3. Alveolar macrophages in alveoli of lungs;
     4. Fixed macrophages/clasmatocytes/histiocytes in skin and subcutaneous tissue
     5. Microglia in brain.
   - A single macrophage can ingest 100 bacteria as well a necrotic material.

3. **Monocytes:** These are actually precursors or immature macrophages and are found in the blood. Once stimulated by the immune system, they are drawn to a needed site (chemotaxis) and migrate through the endothelial lining of the capillary by a process called diapedesis.
   - The monocyte becomes fixed or swells up to five times its original size and becomes a macrophage.
   - Monocytes travel in the blood and are derived in the bone marrow.

4. **Fibrocyte:** Fully differential mature version of a fibroblast.

5. **Adipocyte:** a fixed fat cell (adipose).

6. **Melanocyte:** Stores a brown pigment (melanin).

7. **Mesenchymal Cells:** Stem cells that produce fibroblasts and other connective tissue cells.

8. **Mast Cells:** Large cells found mainly near blood vessels. Mast cells have a dual function: Secrete histamine (vasodilation); Secrete heparin (prevent clotting). Also releases serotonin and bradykinin during inflammation. Work in conjunction with basophils during allergic reactions.

9. **Plasma Cells:** Develop from lymphocytes and are responsible for antibody production.

10. **Lymphocytes:** Derived from lymph tissue, bone marrow, and gut and circulate in blood temporarily before entering lymph system. Eventually go back into the blood and repeat the process.

11. **Red Blood Cells (erythrocytes):** Found in the blood vessels within tissues.

12. **White Blood Cells (leukocytes):** Help remove pathogen toxins, wastes, and damaged cells. There are two classes:
    a. Granular leukocytes including:
       1. Polymorphonuclear neutrophils
       2. Polymorphonuclear esinophils
       3. Polymorphonuclear basophils
    b. Agranular leukocytes including:
       1. Monocytes
       2. Lymphocytes
    - The cells are classified according to their appearance. All granulocytes plus monocytes phagocytize foreign matter. Microscopic lymphocytes attach themselves to a cell and also have an action similar to phagocytes.
    - Another cell classified as a white blood cell, the platelet, is actually a fragment derived from a myeloid stem cell, the magokaryocyte. Platelets help activate the blood clotting mechanism.

13. **Microphages:** A special phagocytizing cell that works closely with a lymphocyte.

CHAPTER 6

THE FIBRILLAR ELEMENTS OF CONNECTIVE TISSUE

The fibrillar elements of connective tissue include twelve different types of collagen, elastin, reticulin, *laminin, fibronectin,* and *chondronectin.*

Some tissues have significant differences in regard to the ratio of cells to extra-cellular material. For example, in bone and muscle, there are high numbers of cells in relation to the extracellular material. In tendons and ligaments, however, the cell number relative to the extracellular material is low. This is because in tendons and ligaments there are only a few number of cells whereas fibrillar components are extensive.

Collagen

Collagen is the connective tissue component best suited to resist tensile forces, in contrast to elastin and reticulin, which have more resiliency and elasticity (Cantu and Grodin 1992). It is composed of an insoluble macromolecule that is helical in design and is extremely adaptable. It can be tough, unyielding, and as rigid as bone, yet, at times, quite pliable (Zohar 1990). Collagen is a remarkably complex group of *glycoproteins* that exists in different forms. In the past, all collagen was believed to be alike, but modern research has identified as many as twelve different types. Of the twelve types of collagen known, types I to IV are most abundant in the body tissues and appear to be most significant for manual therapy.

Collagen is the most common protein in the body, accounting for 40 percent of all protein. In tendons and ligaments, 70 to 90 percent of the dry weight is collagen.

Collagen metabolism is mediated by *morphostasis,* a process that renews both collagen and ground substance. The half-life of collagen is 300 to 500 days in mature, non-traumatized condition. The variation depends on the tissue

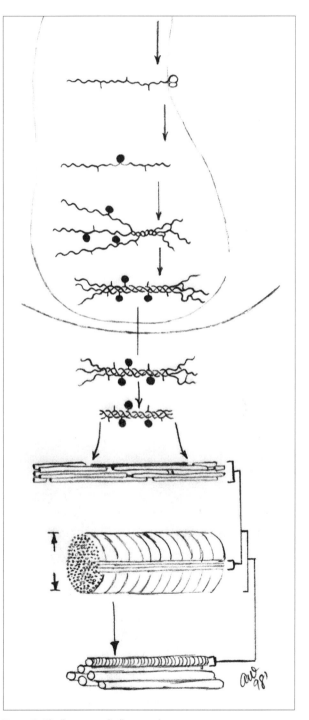

Figure 2. Fibrollogenesis and collagen synthesis.

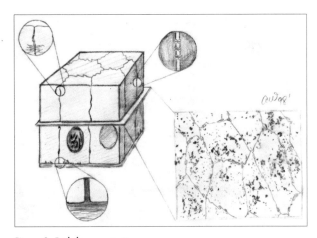

Figure 3. Epithelian organization.

involved, i.e., bones reveal a rapid turnover, while cartilage turns over at a slower rate.

The Origin of Collagen: Fibrillogenesis

The origin of collagen is known as *fibrillogenesis.* The fibroblast cells initiate the production of normal collagen. (See Figures 2 and 3.) Production begins inside the cell. Here, *amino acids* are synthesized into *polypeptide chains* referred to as *procollagen* molecules. These precursors of collagen undergo an enzymatic cleavage of their low molecular weight ends and become *tropocollagen.* Tropocollagen is the functional/structural unit of collagen fibrils. It is the self-assemblage of these *triple helix tropocollagen fibrils* outside the cell that is referred to as fibrillogenesis (Hukins 1984).

After extrusion, *peptides* are cleaved at either end of the procollagen from the cell and molecule. Except in Type IV procollagen, the chains can still undergo considerable transitional changes. These changes occur from either *hydroxylation* or *glycolysation* or both. Such processes lead to modified forms of the same molecule, despite their being coded for by the same gene (Pischinger 1990).

One reason for the inherent strength of the collagen molecule is that the repetition of every third amino acid is *glycine.* Because the glycine molecules are small, they allow collagen to form a tight helix, and this, in turn, translates into greater structural and functional cohesion, similar to a building block. The typical pattern in the collagen chain is X-Y-glycine. "X" and "Y" are, usually, *proline* and *hydroxyproline.* These later two components of amino acids comprise approximately 22 percent of the amino acids. These amino acids can act as stabilizers for the collagen chains via linkage by *disulfide bonds.* Each molecule consists of three separate polypeptide chains that coil into a left handed helix; then the three chains coil together into a right handed superhelix. An additional amino acid that undergoes transition in the collagen molecule is *hydroxylysine.* It is found more in the basement membranes than in the interstitial collagen. Both *lysine* and hydroxylysine undergo transitional reactions that allow for intro- and inter-molecular *cross-linking* (Pischinger 1990).

Once the tropocollagen molecules reach the extracellular space, they arrange themselves in an end-to-end formation, as well as in a parallel, quarter-stacked arrangement. This pattern ensures that one region of the *microfibril* will be no weaker than the other. The fibrils then are bundled together to form large collagen fibers. The fibrils are stable at 37degrees centigrade, but at 40 degrees or above they become unstable and unfold. Individual fibrils occur in periodicities of 67 nm, diameters of approximately 1.5 nm and 280 nm (Hukins 1984). Cross-linking of the parallel fiber alignment adds to the molecules' ability to withstand tensile forces. While molecular attraction creates compactness to each fibril bundle, there exists a minute quantity of clear ground substance separating each strand. (The importance of the ground substance will be discussed later). The three separate polypeptide chains are referred to as *alpha chains.* Combinations of these chains constitute the various types of collagen. Originally these chains were referred to as Alpha I and Alpha II chains, since only one type of collagen was thought to exist (Pischinger 1990). The designations of the chains have been refined as more types of collagen have been discovered.

Each collagen type has slightly different chemical properties. Type I collagen, the most common collagen, consist of two Alpha I (Type I) chains connected to one Alpha I (Type II) chain via a *disulfide bond*. Type I collagen obtains its tensile strength from cross-linking and covalent bonding. These hollow tubules of overlapping molecules have a tensile strength greater than that of steel wire. Cross-linking is tissue specific and based on an adaptation to stress and strain. The cross links also can give way under heavy loads leading to *fibril failure*. Failure begins at 8 to 10 percent strain (Fidone 1975). Type I collagen represents our most abundant component and is found in skin, muscle, tendon, ligament, ordinary loose connective tissue, dense connective tissue, and bone. Modified forms of this collagen containing only Alpha I (Type I) chains have been isolated in a cirrhotic liver, human skin, mouse tumors, and embryonic tendons.

Type II collagen is found primarily in articular cartilage (fibrocartilage and hyaline cartilage). Here the chemical properties consist of three identical alpha chains, with a different amino acid pattern from that in Type I collagen. The three identical chains are referred to as a *trimer* of Alpha I (Type II) chain. This type of collagen exhibits excellent strength qualities without significant flexibility. Type II collagen is actually found in any non-innervated, vascular tissues of the body, including the *intervertebral disc* and the *vitreous humor* of the eye. From these examples, we can see the tremendous versatility of the collagen molecule. As the Type I collagen molecule mixes with hyaline, which is a nylon-like substance from the *chondroblast*, the resultant tissue becomes a buffer for joint compression, friction, and movement. Hyaline cartilage exhibits the tensile strength of steel. In the second example, this type of collagen in the *cornea* is as transparent as glass, yet it can become as tenacious as glue, as

viscous as gelatin, or as diffuse as water (Zohar 1990).

Type III generally has smaller fibrils and fewer cross-links than Type I and II (Hollinshead 1985). Type II collagen is typically found deposited in tissue repair and is replaced later by molecularly larger Type I collagen. An excessive amount of Type II collagen actually weakens Type II chains (Hollinshead 1985). Type III differs chemically from Type I and II in that it contains *cystine* in two adjacent positions at the junction between the helical and non-helical *carboxy terminal peptides* (Hollinshead 1985). The triple helix is held together by disulfide bonds which help decrease the propensity towards *collagenase degradation*. Although found in conjunction with the larger, Type I collagen, Type III collagen's functional nature is seen in tissues that require a modicum of flexibility. Such tissues include the skin, aorta, other blood vessels, lungs, fetal skin, synovia, uterus, fascia, ligaments, and placental tissues (Cantu and Grodin 1992; Pischinger 1990; Hollinshead 1985). Type III collagen within ligaments offers extensibility but not elasticity in regards to stretch. This is important to the manual therapist, as the stability of this collagen will affect its *viscoelastic* nature. This means that once a load is placed on the tissue and over-stretching occurs, the increased length remains after the load is removed.

Type IV collagen is not as abundant as the first three types, nor is it similar in regards to its chemical composition. Chemically, Type IV collagen or *basement membrane collagen*, as it is sometimes called, doesn't have a typical 67 nm periodicity and is much more heavily glycosylated (Hollinshead 1985). Two structurally different Alpha chains combine to create Type IV collagen: Alpha I Type IV and Alpha II Type IV molecule chains. These chains have a less stable structure than the helical design of collagen Types I to III. As a basement membrane, the collagen is not present in the form of fibrils but is organized into a net-like structure (Pischinger 1990; Hollinshead

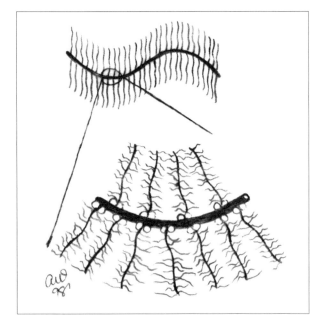

Figure 4. Proteoglycan arrangement.

1985). Basement membranes actually act as support layers for the cells that cover various body surfaces (epithelium), hence, connective tissues are never exposed to an outside environment.

Other collagen includes Type V collagen, a pericellular tissue whose typical chemical make-up is Alpha I Type V and Alpha II Type V chains in a 2:1 ratio, while other molecules have been identified as having Alpha 3 Type V chains in addition to the two latter forms. This collagen, with a 1:1:1 ratio is best isolated in the uterus. Type V collagen has been found in the *placental villi* and skin. It never comprises more than 10 percent of the total collagen in any tissue.

Type VI collagen has a close association with Type V collagen and has also been isolated in the skin, uterus, placental villi, and *synovia*. The Type VI collagen chain consists of Alpha I Type IV, Alpha II Type VI, and Alpha III Type VI molecules (Martini 1989.)

As more collagen type tissues are discovered within our cellular milieu, greater understanding of their significance will also be found. There are another six types of collagen already isolated in the body; surely more will follow! The reasons for differentiation are not clearly understood. The number of type of collagen dictates its significance.

Elastin

A basic fibrillar component in the extra-cellular matrix is elastin. Elastin is found in the skin, tendon, *ligmentum nuchae, ligmentum flavum*, lungs, and linings of arteries. It is more elastic than collagen proper. Pischinger notes that the elastin precursor tropoelastin contains an amino acid tetrapeptide that includes: glycine, *valine*, proline, and glycine repetitive sequences. Since elastin is insoluble, the tropoelastin soluble precursor is used to extrapolate a model. Secondary to high glycine and hydroxyproline content, it has been thought that elastin develops from collagen. These fibers react to stress and strain along the lines and direction of forces and are able to recoil to their original shape when a stretch is released. Elastin has been likened to a rubber band because of its recoil capability. There is an order of molecular chains associated with entropy loss during stretching, which is then regained when the stretch is removed. Whether this actually occurs in elastin is a matter of conjecture; it does represent a plausible model. Elastin is by comparison a much smaller microfibrillar network than collagen fibers. The resiliency of these fibers changes when the temperature drops; elastin can actually become brittle at 20 degrees centigrade. When ligaments are observed under a microscope, it is common to observe elastin extensibility by a built-in crimp within the layers of the parallel fibers. (See Figure 4.)

Under stress loads, the elastin molecule straightens and takes on a more collagen-like function while increasing its tensile characteristics. Peripheral ligaments have relatively little elastin, whereas the intervertebral disc is an excellent example of a tissue type with large amounts of it. Elastic fiber ratios in other tissue differ significantly. The range is from 1 to 5 percent (dry weight) in skin, loose connective tissue and tendons, to 50 percent (dry weight) in elastic arteries. The *tunica media* of the human aorta, for example, have 50 to 60 elastic membranes arranged concentrically and separated by 6 to 18 nm of connective tissue spaces filled with extra-cellular matrix. The layers are approximately 2.5 nm thick. As well as being resilient, elastin fibers are known to be unaffected by acids, alkalis, or heat.

Reticulin

Reticulin fibers comprise another glycoprotein that is less tensile than either collagen or elastin. There is a slight variation in the combination of protein subunit sequences within this tissue. As its name implies, this tissue forms networks that weave and interlock, allowing for a durable yet pliable meshing. It is a delicate tissue that is found in and around the internal organs and glands. Reticulin exhibits the same periodicity as colla-gen. It has also been found to contain Type II col-lagen and fibronectin.

Fibronectin

One of the more recent molecular discoveries is fibronectin. It was first recognized on the cell sur-face, then as a tissue adhesive, and most recently as a constituent of blood plasma. It is a network forming glycoprotein that is synthesized by many structures, including red blood cells, lymphocytes, neutrophils, macrophages, basophils and esino-phils. Fibronectin apparently has functions which allow for intra- and extracellular communication regarding homeostatis.

Laminin

Laminin is another network-forming glycopro-tein that is connected with basement membrane adhesion to the epithelia (Type IV collagen).

Chondronectin

Chondronectin is yet another network-forming glycoprotein that is associated with adhesion fac-tors for chondrocytes and Type II collagen.

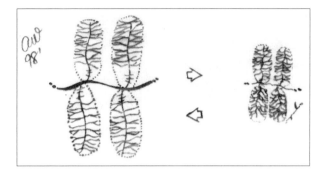

Figure 5. Proteoglycan compression.

Ground Substance

The ground substance is the environment in which all connective tissue components exist (See Table III and Figure 5.) As mentioned previously, the fibroblast, a specialized cell from the mesoderm and the mast cell, produces most of the elements of connective tissue including the ground sub-stance. This is the non-fibrous component of the connective tissue matrix. Although the composi-tion of the ground substance varies from tissue to tissue, several core components and functions are repeated in all environments. It is found in all the body's connective tissue, but it is distinctly different from tissue fluid. The other intercellu-lar fluids seep from capillaries and tissue cells and exist within the ground substance. These other fluids are in need of the ground substance for cer-tain activities to occur (Fitton-Jackson 1965). Specifically, the ground substance provides a bar-rier against invading bacteria and other organ-isms; it allows for a diffusion of waste products and nutrients from the vascular structures; and it helps maintain the critical fiber distance between collagen fibers. This latter function helps prevent micro adhesions, provides tissue volume, and maintains extensibility.

The primary components of the ground sub-stance are *glycosaminoglycans (GAGs)* and water. GAGs are *polysaccharides* (formerly called *acid mucopolysaccharides*) where two linked sugars are chemically repeated (Rich 1975). (See Figures 3 and 6.) These GAGs not only perform the

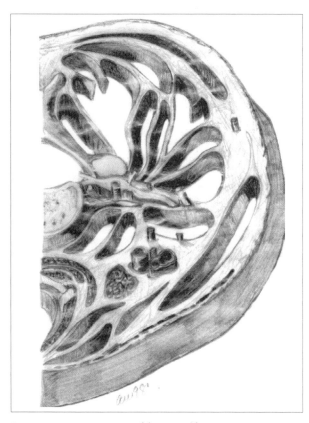

Figure 6. Transverse cross-section of deep cervical fascia.

previously listed functions but also have a lubricating effect on tissues. Large polysaccharides called *proteoglycans* are covalently attached to a protein and a glycoprotein. The glycoproteins are large proteins attached to a polysaccharide. The proteoglycans bind with water (approximately 70 percent of total connective tissue content) and form one of the largest molecular aggregates in the body. They are linked with the function of *hyaluronic acid* and, among other functions, give cartilage some of its viscoelastic properties (Rich 1975).

GAGs are separated into sulfated groups (that include *chondroitin sulfate, dermatan sulfate, heparin sulfate, keratan sulfate*) and non-sulfated groups inclusive of hyaluronic acid. Chondroitin sulfate contributes to the rigidity of the ground substance in cartilage; hyaluronic acid, as stated above, binds with water. Because of its binding capacity with water, hyaluronic acid is found in many tissues, especially those that are soft and gel-like, for instance, the vitreous humor of the eye. Chondroitin sulfate, on the other hand, is found in bone, skin, arterial walls, and cartilage. Keratan sulfate is found in skin, tendon, heart valves, and blood vessels. The variation of the consistency of the ground substance ranges from a viscous gel to a watery gel state, depending on the properties required at different locations.

The ground substance permeates the entire body's tissues to the level of the cell and is closely aligned with all of the systems activities. It is a facilitator as well as a barrier between cellular substances and blood (Lowen 1990). Any alteration of these functions through trauma, stress or strain, fatigue, malnutrition or build up of toxic materials can lead to a breakdown of the body's chemical and physical equilibrium. For instance, if the lymphatic system were completely shut down, death would occur within approximately twenty-four hours due to cellular toxicity. Lymph, lymph tissue, and vessels are all connective tissue derivatives, and the ground substance is a significant transit element in the loose connective tissue in the *interstitium*. In other words, the ground substance is not the inert substance it was once thought to be. On the contrary, it is a variable factory of activity that actually represents a common link between all branches of medicine (Boone 1996).

As noted above, ground substance is distributed extensively throughout the body. It significantly influences the body's physiologic processes as well as the body's potential for pathology. The ground substance is in a constant state of flux via metabolic changes. Within the tendon, ligament, and bone tissues, the ground substance is referred to as the *matrix*.

Even though the ground substance comprises the immediate environment of every cell in the body, there are still barriers to its influence, for instance, between blood and organ tissue (parenchyma). This physiochemical barrier has several parameters, specifically, the *cell membrane, interstitial fluid* (both components), reticuloendothelial tissue and capillary membrane.

The authors wish to point out that the ground substance is the key environment on which to focus for attaining a multiplanar myofascial release. This is more important than focusing on the viscoelastic components of connective tissue. Too much emphasis has been placed on the viscoelastic components.

To maintain the homeostatic mechanisms within the body it is necessary to maintain the health and function of the connective tissue components.

The regulation of connective tissue metabolism is not achieve by any single factor. The fluctuating equilibrium within the body's tissues is greatly affected by the regional diversity of cells within the connective tissue. *Protein messengers* called *mediators* allow for intercellular regulation. The cell manufactures the mediators and, as of the time of this writing, over 300 of them have been identified. Examples include: histamine, prostaglandin, bradykinin, and leukotrienes.

Beyond these manufactured mediators, the by-products of activity within the ground substance can actually act as their own mediators. In general, the mediators can take on various functions; they can interact with other mediators that are secondary to the activity at any particular cell site. Mediators can also act like tissue barriers, keeping certain organisms out of an area where they don't belong and holding others in where they do. Under normal conditions, mediators collectively help to maintain tissue equilibrium. Under abnormal or pathologic conditions these same mediators can be injurious to the tissues. For example, prostaglandins are needed to protect the stomach lining from excessive acid corrosion; yet in a situation where too much of it is synthesized by the cell, a different intervention may be required to offset that over-production. Specific mediators possessing anabolic and catabolic qualities govern the microhomeostasis between the cell and the matrix (Weiss 1984).

Table III
Extracellular Matrix Components

Fibers-Glycoproteins

1. Collagen: Protein substrate in a repeating sequence of three units. Stiff but pliable molecules with high tensile strength and poor stretch capability. There are over twelve types of collagen, but four types are most important: Type I, found in loose and dense connective tissue proper; Type II, found in cartilage; Type III, found in arteries and fetal dermas; Type IV, found at the level of the basement membrane.

2. Elastin: Elastin is a protein that affords extensive tissue flexibility. Tissue itself can be stretched up to 130 percent of its initial length. It has perfect recoil capabilities.

3. Fibronectin: Along with laminin and chondonectin, this constitutes a network of glycoproteins, an important constituent of blood plasma that is synthesized by many cell types including: red blood cells, lymphocytes, fibrocytes, basophils, neutraphils, esinophils, and macrophages.

4. Reticulin: Composed of reticular fibers that form a meshwork that is flexible yet durable. These tissues have the same protein sequences as collagen with slight pattern variations. This tissue is found predominantly in the viscera, i.e., spleen and liver.

5. Laminin: Network-forming glycoprotein that is connected to the basement membrane and adhesion to the epithelial layers. (Type IV collagen)

6. Chondronectin: Network forming glycoprotein that is associated with adhesion factors for chondrocytes and Type II collagen and cartilage.

Ground Substance

A saline gel that permeates and surrounds cells throughout the entire organism. It is composed of several macromolecules.

1. Proteoglycan: A sugar protein complex with an electric charge suitable for extensive water binding capabilities. Proteoglycans can be either monomers or aggregates. Glycosaminoglycans attach to the protein backbone which links with hyaluronic acid molecules.

2. Glycosaminoglycans (GAGs): Referred to as mucopolysaccharides in older research. Composed of sulfated and non-sulfated disaccharide units including chondroitin sulfate, dematan sulfate, hyaluronic acid, heparan suflate, and keratin sulfate. The GAGs represent building blocks for proteoglycan molecules. Functionally, they help maintain the critical fiber distance thus inhibiting dysfunctional cross-linking among some fibers.

CHAPTER 7

THE PROTECTIVE FUNCTION OF MUSCLE: TENSEGRITY

The Protective Function of Muscle

In the not too distant past, bone was considered, qua tissue, as an insignificant, even inert, body tissue that acted merely as a spacer for musculo-tendonous and ligament attachments. As a result of new clinical information, new directions in assessment and treatment of bone pathology are being developed almost on a daily basis. This information comes from recognizing new applications of "old" information, from original research, and from the creation of new and unique rehabilitative constructs.

In a similar fashion, our understanding of the function of muscle tissue has undergone a drastic revision. Muscle, for example, has essentially always been identified with its movement capability. Moving a person or body part from one place to another has been seen as its primary function. In our clinics and seminars, we have undertaken a closer look at an alternate function of muscle: its protective function. We have recognized the monumental importance of this function and how in most clinical situations its presence takes precedence over any considerations of movement. For example, consider the phenomenon of protective muscle spasm. In addition to being subjectively uncomfortable, a spasm can serve the interests of the organism, for example, under conditions of trauma by limiting range of motion, splinting a joint, and protecting against unwanted movement, all on a lower motor neuron level! Thanks to our awareness of this, we have applied basic neurologic constructs and self-protective patterns to upper motor neuron problems and found that the body can, and often does, have distinct mechanics at the higher spinal cord, brain stem, and cortex that require the maximum protection after injury. In other words, once we applied our lower motor neuron concepts to upper motor neuron problems such as stroke, cerebral palsy, and TBIs, we were able to facilitate major changes in structure and function. Addressing the muscle's protective function first, before its movement function, leads to far more dramatic changes than the other way around.

We see this protective function of muscles in many different areas. Skeletal and smooth muscle protection is evident within and beyond the boundaries of many systems including the nerves, bones, blood vessels, joints, and viscera. From our clinical research we have observed, monitored, and treated smooth muscle spasm at the level of *lymphatic chains, vascular constriction* of both veins and arteries, and *viscero-spasm* secondary to *ulcers, colitis,* and *hernias.* The list of problems and pathologies that we are able to address using this approach is extensive and continues to grow.

The function of protection occurs automatically, autonomically and instantaneously in most cases. (Weiselfish) Giammatteo and colleagues have been focusing not only on the clinical significance of this phenomenon for over ten years at the time of this writing, but also on the structural and functional sequelae of the protective activities. (Weiselfish) Giammatteo has localized over 600 individual and specific pathoanatomic dysfunctions classified as *compression syndromes.* These syndromes have been found to occur within and between systems. No tissue is immune to dysfunction. It has become more apparent to us with each clinical case we examine, that the body's ability to self-protect is as great or even greater than the body's ability to heal itself. Each presentation must be acknowledged and assessed carefully to see if its etiology involves the protective mechanism. Even our "learned" movement patterns serve as much as a developmental reflection of these core protective mechanisms as they do of our neural developmental processes.

Tensegrity

Many practitioners within the field of rehabilitation are familiar with the basic constructs of myofascial release techniques. An underacknowledged concept presented by Ingber and Juhan may add a broader base of understanding to the whole spectrum of connective tissue literature. The concept of tensegrity or "tensional integrity" has extensive applications to our use of connective tissue bio- physiology and mechanics. The term "tensegrity" was coined by Buckminster Fuller to describe a natural phenomena whereby a "system stabilizes itself mechanically via an intricate balance and distribution of compressional and tensional forces on the skeleton." Ingber's research and application expanded our understanding of this concept.

First of all, Ingber (Ingber 1998) noted a consistent organizational pattern of tissues with a well-defined hierarchy at every level of body tissue. He also noted that these same tissues exhibit a similar pattern of self-assembly from the smallest cellular levels to the largest organ or system levels in the body. Within this consistent, contiguous, and continuous framework is the architectural design of tensegrity. Ingber and Juhan agree definitionally that tensegrity "refers to a system that stabilizes itself mechanically through a balance of tension and compressive forces." FN Ingber notes that the self-stabilization phenomena can be exhibited on all levels: microscopic to macroscopic. Clinically, this has excellent applications, especially to the 3-Planar Myofascial Fulcrum techniques. In other words, the existence of tensional and compressive balance not only exists at the level of the muscles, fascia, tendons, and ligaments, but more importantly it also has been seen at the molecular level, i.e., proteins, carbohydrates, fats and even extracellular matrix.

Specifically, Ingber showed that cells contain an internal framework of protein polymers that he referred to as *cyotoskeleton*. He was able to simulate how a finite network of contractile microfilaments actually extends through the cell, pulling the contents towards the cell nucleus. He localized additional forces within the cell as well as within the extracellular matrix that work in opposition-of-balance stress on the cell. Adhesion receptors on the cell surface known as *integrins* help transmit these forces from the external to the internal milieu of the cell. Ingber realized the profound implications of the tensegrity model. He stated that "the existence of a force balance was a way to provide a means to integrate mechanics and biochemistry at the molecular level" FN Secondary to the tensegrity design, he found it possible to change the cell cytoskeleton by altering the balance of physical forces transmitted across the cell surface. This finding is important because many of the enzymes and other substances that control protein synthesis, energy conversion, and growth in the cell are physically immobilized on the cyotoskeleton. For this reason, changing cytoskeletal geometry and mechanics could affect biochemical reactions and even alter the genes that are activated and thus the proteins that are made. Ingber even noted that depending on the type of stress induction to the cell surface, reactions were stimulated at a cellular level.

The profound clinical implications of tensegrity can best be seen when examining our fascial fulcrum concept. By introducing minimally maintained stresses in specific patterns, we can transduce forces to the level of the cell and theoretically affect its functional capacity. Ingber's research can easily be extrapolated to both treatment techniques and potential outcomes. If we can change cyotoskeleton configurations through force transmission from an external myofascial fulcrum, we should have an increased potential for affecting a multitude of pathological conditions. In other words, we step beyond a pathomechanical model to a pathophysiological or pathochemical model.

Application of this concept with our clinical skills may well explain why we have had excellent outcomes with medical conditions heretofore not addressed in this manner. These include diabetes mellitus, spinal cord injury, stroke, multiple sclerosis, cancer, radiation sequelae, attention deficit disorder, autism, pervasive developmental disorder, infection, immune system suppression, traumatic brain injury, migraines, carpal tunnel syndrome, visceral dysfunction, infertility, scarring, and amyotrophic lateral sclerosis, to name just a few.

Juhan's and especially Ingber's insights, when combined in a functional, clinical, and practical approach, lend significant validity and objectivity to a theoretical concept that has largely been based on conjecture and subjectivity to date.

CHAPTER 8
STRUCTURE AND FUNCTION ON A TISSUE LEVEL

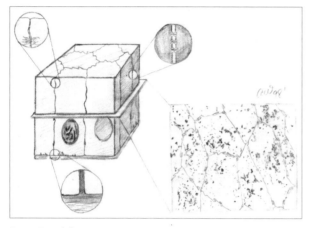

Figure 7. Epithelian organization.

As an introduction to the complex and encompassing nature of the body's connective tissue, a review of its intimate relationships with other primary tissue types is required. As stated earlier, the four basic tissue types are: (1) epithelial tissue, (2) connective tissue, (3) muscle tissue and (4) nerve tissue. Connective tissue comprises approximately 45 percent of the total volume of the body, muscle tissue accounts for approximately 50 percent, nerve and epithelial tissues together consist of the remaining 5 percent. Considering the large volume of connective tissue, one would expect considerable clinical attention to the assessment and treatment of these tissues. This in fact is happening within the allopathic profession, as is evidenced by the recent increase of diagnoses such as *fibrositis, myofibrosities* and *fibromyalgia*.

After a brief look at the nature of epithelial tissue, in this chapter we will discuss the main categories of connective tissue and their subdivisions.

Epithelial Tissue

The epithelial tissues cover exposed surfaces and line internal structures that directly and indirectly have a connection to the external environment (Weiss 1984). In other words, these cells form layers that act as *barriers* not only to external forces, but to internal influences as well. The epithelium is partially held together by proteoglycans, a sort of intercellular cement (Weiss 1984). While the cells are packed together tightly with an outer surface always exposed to the external environment and an inner surface attached to the basement membrane. This membrane is divided into two parts. The first is the *basal lamina* which contains glycoproteins and protein filaments. The second, deeper part is the *reticular lamina* which contains protein fibers and whose genesis is from connective tissue cells. (See Figure 4.)

While the reticular lamina gives this membrane its strength, the basal lamina provides a functional barrier that inhibits material from connective tissue anchoring into the epithelium. The epithelial tissues not only provide physical protection and permeability screening for underlying structures; but they also provide sensory capabilities, i.e., pain and touch receptors in the skin. They also produce secretions from specialized gland cells. *Exocrine secretions* are released on the surface of the epithelial tissues, while *endocrine secretions* (hormones) permeate the cells, enter the blood system, and influence various target organs (Calliet 1988). Epithelia are classified according to their layers and shapes. There is current recognition of various shapes and at least two different layers. No matter epithelia are classified, however, the schema must show that connective tissue underlies the basement membrane, which in turn is covered by epithelia, so that the connective tissues are never exposed to the external environment.

Connective Tissue

Connective tissues vary in location, function, and structure. All connective tissues derive from the embryonic mesenchyme and then assume distinctive gross and microscopic features and subserve a variety of functions.

The connective tissues are categorized by several types and subtypes. The first type is *connective tissue proper,* also referred to as *ordinary connective tissue.* Each of these is in turn is divided into two subgroups: *loose connective tissue* and *dense connective tissue.* There is yet a further delineation of form for each of these subdivisions: some researchers note a regular or irregular arrangement of fibers (Boone 1996). This will be expanded upon later.

The second type of connective tissue is *supporting connective tissue* and includes bone and cartilage. The third type of connective tissue, with a distinct make-up, is *fluid connective tissue.* It includes blood and lymph.

The physical and biomechanical properties of the fibers together with the ground substance contribute to the nature of the matrix. Some collagen arrangements of fibers appear in parallel (for example, ligaments and tendons) while scar tissue and dermis exhibit a fibrous, irregular arrangement. *Elastic tissues* have a predominance of elastin fibers and *adipose tissue,* which is mostly connective tissue infiltrated by fat cells.

Connective Tissue Proper

Loose Connective Tissue

Loose connective tissue or *areolar tissue* exists as a fine cobweb-like packing material—a padding that fills the interstices between the organs. It is also found between the dermis and the underlying structures, i.e., muscle or bone, and over body parts that are devoid of subcutaneous fat, such as the *dorsum* of the hand. The loose connective tissue underlying the skin and infiltrated with adipose tissue is found in *superficial fascia.* This tissue helps conserve body heat and is responsible for body contours. The loose connective tissue has an open framework, and the ground substance accounts for most of its volume. Because the fiber arrangement is loose and there is a large fluid content, this tissue is able to distort without significant damage. The addition of elastic fibers allows for further absorption of shock, as well as excellent recoil capabilities. There is an expansive circulatory supply in the tissue that helps facilitate the quick uptake of medication, the delivery of oxygen and nutrients, and the removal of carbon dioxyde and waste products. The loose connective tissue can also help with diffusion across the epithelial membrane in order to provide oxygen and nutrients to the cells.

Fascia

Fascia is yet another delineation of the body's connective tissue specialization. At times it is difficult to distinguish fascia from loose connective tissue or from other body structures. Descriptions of fascia are at times confusing because of the layer effect exhibited by the tissue within enclosing or surrounding systems. An example of this is the fascial specialization in the *tunica adventitia* for example or the *tunica externa,* i.e., the outer layer of the blood vessels—which blend in with the surrounding loose connective tissue that acts as an anchor for the circulatory vessel. A similar phenomenon occurs for muscle and nerve connective tissue layering.

Microscopically, fascia differs from loose connective tissue by its greater quantity of collagen fibers. Fascial fibers are much more organized than those of loose connective tissue but less so than the collagen found in tendons, ligaments, and aponeuroses. Macroscopically, there are two distinct fascial systems: one lines the thoracic and abdominal cavities; the second is the external, or investing fascia, which lies deep to the *tela subcutanea,* the deep fascia. The internal fasciae which line the thoracic cavity and the abdominal cavity are referred to as *endothoracic* and *endoabdominal* fascia. These barely discernible linings

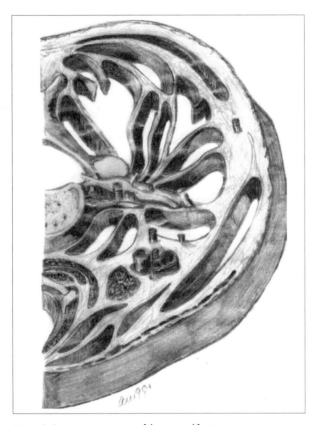

Figure 8. Transverse cross-section of deep cervical fascia.

affix the parietal layer of the *serous sacs,* the *pleura* in the thorax, and the *peritoneum* in the abdomen, to the inner aspect of the body wall (Kain 1996). Loose connective tissue is usually not included as part of the internal fascia category, even though the *endopelvic fascia,* a continuation of the endoabdominal fascia, is actually specialized loose connective tissue. Other specializations exist within these layers, such as the *suprapleural membrane.* This is a thickening of the endothoracic fascia over the dome of the lung. Unlike these specializations, the internal fascia has regional identifications based on the muscles it contacts; for instance the *transverse fascia, psoas fascia,* and *diaphragmatic fascia* (Calliet 1988). The psoas fascia, on the right side of the body, is merely a continuation in part from *Toldts' fascia* which anchors the ascending colon. Specialized regional anatomy and its functional significance will be covered later in this text.

Once the tela subcutaneous (superficial fascia) is removed, the deep tissues are dominated by collagen fibers. These are referred to as dense connective tissue and elastic tissue. The regular dense connective tissue consists of tendons, ligaments, and fascia, while elastic tissue is found between the vertebrae of the spine. Dense irregular connective tissue is best illustrated in the dermis of the skin and capsules of some organs. These tissues provide stabilization, reduce friction, provide attachments, absorb shock, improve alignment, and resist movement in many directions.

The example of the deep cervical fascia illustrates an aspect of this tissue's adaptability. (See Figure 8.) In the neck and limbs, the deep fascia is a tough fibrous connective tissue layer that surrounds the particular body part. From its deep roots it sends septa into and among many muscles. In the back of the arm, the deep fascia is fused to the surface of the muscle, while in the front of the arm it forms a loosely fitting envelope around the muscle. Where greater function and separation of structure is needed, such as by the cervical spine, the fascial layers become more refined, definitive and intricate (Barral 1993).

Regional demands on connective tissue, for example, stress and strain, are exemplified nicely by those made by ligaments and tendons. Skeletal ligaments are distinct kinds of connective tissue that traverse joints and, at times, blend into the fibrous walls of the joint cavity or capsule. It is often suggested that ligaments "hold joints together." This would lead one to believe that ligaments have contractile tissue. In actuality, the ligaments keep joints from coming part. The authors suggest that ligaments have a role in the coordination of neighboring bones, as well as a larger guidance role of the body and person.

Heavier ligaments sometimes resemble tendons, as in the case of the *infrapatellar ligament*. It is actually a continuation of the tendinous extension from the *quadriceps* that is interrupted by the *patellar tendon* (Kain 1996). *Visceral ligaments* vary in tensile strength depending upon the motility and mobility of an organ (Barral 1993). The stomach, for example, has a strong attachment to the diaphragm: the *gastrophrenic ligament*. Other ligaments that connect to the stomach, e.g., the *lesser omentum*, are actually part of the *mesentery*, a thin sheet of connective tissue with mesothelial surfaces that conduct blood and lymph vessels and nerves to other structures. These attachments are more functional than structural in nature. The left and right *triangular ligaments* and the two leaves of the *coronary ligament* anchoring the liver are modified mesenteries that have more of a supportive function (Kain 1996). As the connective tissue, ligaments, fascia, and loose connective tissue are viewed from the upper abdominal cavity to the pelvic floor, an increased regional thickening is noticeable farther away from the diaphragm. In other words, more passive support of the lower organs is needed for the inferior abdominal contents. This is partially due to the decreasing effects of the sub-atmospheric pressure from the thoracic cavity on the caudal organs and structures (Weiselfish 1981; Berquist 1978).

Some ligaments are actually remnants of parts of the fetus that are no longer utilized as they were in utero, e.g., the *medial umbilical ligaments* are formed from the *umbilical arteries*. There are ligaments that contain smooth muscle or are formed largely from them, e.g., the *ligament of Trietz* is also referred to as the *suspensory muscle of the duodenal jejunal junction* (Barral 1993).

Tendons are continuations into bones of the superficial fascial layers of muscle, as noted previously, and are usually inert. They are continuous with the periosteum. In some instances, the tendon blends with the dense connective tissue that forms the deep layer of the skin (*corium* or *dermis*) (Kain 1996). Tendons insert over bony prominences, thus, either a bursa or a *tendon sheath* protects the connective tissue. Tendon sheaths are connective tissue layers that split and form a cavity that surrounds the tendon.

The external surface is the visceral layer, while the internal layer surrounding the cavity is the *parietal layer*. The two layers are continuous through a *mesotendon;* which a thin film of fluid separates. In some areas, cartilage or bone, i.e., *sesamoids,* develop within tendons where excessive friction is too great for the bursa or sheathing. Bursas are usually developed before birth, but can develop in adulthood in response to friction (Kain 1996).

Supporting Connective Tissue

Cartilage

Classified as a supporting connective tissue, cartilage provides static and dynamic supporting structures for the rest of the body's systems. A significant feature is its avascular nature. (See Figure 9.) The matrix of cartilage contains *chondrocytes*. These negate the formation of blood vessels. Proteoglycan chondroitin sulfate comprises the gel that is the signature of cartilage.

Cartilage is divided into three types: *fibrocartilage, hyaline cartilage,* and *elastic cartilage.* Fibrocartilage is found in several places in the body, especially in the intervertebral disc. It is also found in some weight bearing joints, e.g., knee, pelvis, lower jaw, and ends of the clavicles.

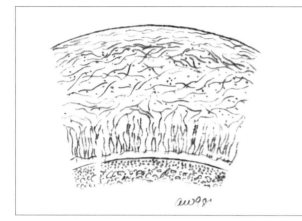

Figure 9. Organization of articular cartilage.

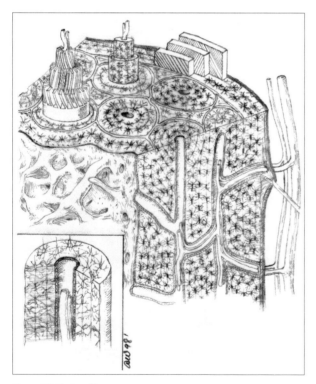

Figure 10. Section of bone.

Hyaline cartilage is found in the cartilage of the ribs, the rings that support the *trachea* and its branches, and the surfaces of bones within joints. Elastic cartilage is found only in the external ear, the lower part of the nose, and the *epiglottis* (Valliet 1988; Lowen 1990; Kain 1996).

Fluid Connective Tissue

Blood and Lymph Cells

Blood and lymph cells are classified as fluid connective tissues (Lowen 1990). (See Figure 1.) *Erythrocytes* (red blood cells) account for over half of the blood's volume. The fluid matrix of blood is the plasma that contains other cellular elements important for immune system function, i.e., monocytes and leukocytes. Interstitial fluid and lymph exist along with the plasma in the extracellular environment of the cell. Plasma and interstitial fluid amounts vary based on concentrations of dissolved proteins (Fitton-Jackson 1965). Lymph represents the true waste disposal system of the body, with 99 percent of available cells being lymphocytes, as well as microphages and macrophages.

Bone

Bone is another modification of supporting connective tissue. (See Figure 10.) Whereas chondrocytes are the dominant cell in cartilage, *osteocytes* are bone's number one building block. Collagen has an extraordinary relationship in bone with both *calcium phosphate* and *calcium carbonate*. Isolated, the calcium salts are brittle but strong, and the collagen fibers are comparatively weak but flexible. Together they create a tissue that has phenomenal tensile strength, similar to steel-reinforced concrete (Lowen 1990). Bones remain one of the body's highest metabolically active structures. They are no longer considered an inert tissue (Proctor 1977). Another important characteristic of this tissue is its ability to effect complete repair in the case of an injury, whereas avascular cartilage has limited potential for the like.

Tissue Spaces

Tissue spaces are filled with *extracellular fluid*. The spaces act as a medium for interchange between cells, blood, and *lymphatics*. These spaces are products of loose connective tissue interstices, i.e., space between the fibers. Fascial spaces are found among the deep layers of connective tissue. These spaces are usually described as loose connective tissues that lie between muscles, or are bound by connective tissue layers dense enough to be called fascia. Fluid, blood, and pus can accumulate here (Kain 1996).

CHAPTER 9

CONNECTIVE TISSUE AND DEVELOPMENTAL DIFFERENTIATION

The ground substance has the ability to alter its consistency from gel to solution and back again, depending on the needs of the immediate environment. (See Figure 4.) When this substance is thought of in combination with collagen of varying densities and amounts and with specialized cells, the ubiquitous nature of connective tissue can be recognized. The differentiation of ground substance within bone, cartilage, tendon, muscle, nerve, vessels, ligaments, and organs is specialized and unique to each tissue. Examination of many of these tissues will provide the practitioner with a better understanding of the variety and expansiveness, as well as the extensive nature of connective tissue. Connective tissue in all its forms, specialized and otherwise structured, is continuous and contiguous throughout the entire body. It extends from just beneath the skin to the deep fascia which connect to and through the periosteum. There are specific connective tissue connections in the cranium and spinal column, including the dura of the spinal cord and deeper cord tissues (Lowen 1992). Further clarifications of the body's fascial sheaths will be discussed in accordance with topographic divisions.

The manual practitioner can affect essentially all of the connective tissues, either directly or indirectly, with the techniques described later in this text. The close examination of several of these specific tissues in the present chapter will facilitate our analysis of histological and biomechanical components.

Bones represent the maximally gelled state of connective tissue. (See Figure 10.) Once considered merely structural rigging for muscles and ligaments, bone is now considered one of the most metabolically active structures of the body (Berquist 1978). Bone is derived from the mes-

enchyme, which is the tissue responsible for the development of the collagen molecule and other closely related structures, e.g., muscle, blood cartilage and lymph, etc. Bone is also comprised of both organic and inorganic components. A high content of mineral salts combine with an organic matrix. These minerals, consisting of calcium and phosphate, are also referred to as *hydroxyapatite crystals*. The mineral crystals provide a harness for bone, similar to sedimentary rock. The collagen fibers give bone its flexibility and elastic resiliency. The mineral content of bones comprises only 75 percent of living bone, the remaining 25 percent consisting of connective tissue, inclusive of the ground substance. Collagen accounts for approximately 95 percent of the extracellular ,i.e., organic component of bone (Hukins 1984). The ground substance consists of glycosaminoglycans, which serves as a cementing material for the mineralized collagen fibers. This latter substance constitutes approximately 5 percent of the total weight of the bone. There are, in addition, small amounts of *carbonate* within the organic matrix. The combination of the inorganic and organic components of bone creates a material that resists compression, torsion, shearing, dislocation, and bending. The two components together form a functional relationship that excedes the strength of each component alone. It has been said that "bone can compete with the best steel-reinforced concrete, at a considerable savings in weight." (Lowen 1990). Simply put, the combination of collagen and hydroxyapatite crystals offers us a true "flexible solid."

The building blocks of bone, as previously stated, begin with the mesenchymal tissue. Some of this tissue differentiates into *osteoblasts* that help lay down the matrix of bone. These cells then further differentiate into *osteocytes,* which are an integral histological component in the *Haversian Canal System,* the basic functional unit of bones. The concentric layers of calcified matrix known as *lamellae* are permeated with small channels called *caniculi.* These allow the vasculature and extensions of the osteocytes vital interconnections for the diffusion of waste. They also provide nutrients to the other aspects of bone (Lowen 1990).

The outer layer of bone is covered by periosteum, a dense fibrous tissue that is infiltrated by blood and nerve vessels, with connections to the Haversian Canal System. The periosteum has the additional function of bone repair and growth. The periosteum is continuous with the collagen of the *joint capsule,* as well as with many tendinous insertions (Hukins 1984). Although the periosteum blends with the joint capsule, it doesn't cover the ends of bones at joint surfaces. This is reserved for articular cartilage. An inner cellular layer of the periosteum is referred to as the *endosteum.* It is active during growth, repair, and remodeling (Lowen 1990).

From a fluid connective tissue viewpoint, it is easy to recognize the importance of maintaining the sol (solution) state of the ground substance of bone and its continual balance within the inorganic component. Bone not only serves as a support mechanism for the soft tissues and organs. It also acts in several other capacities: as a storage compartment for lipids and important mineral reserves; as an important energy reserve; as a producer of red blood cells in its red marrow. Additionally, it serves as static and dynamic protector of softer structures within the body and as a lever system for varying mechanical advantages (Lowen 1990). The health and maintenance of the structure and function of bone can be traced directly to the connective tissue components housed within the solid framework of this multifaceted system.

Cartilage

Another type of supportive connective tissue is cartilage. (See Figure 9.) Unlike the osteocytes in bone, cartilage is made up of a matrix of chondrocytes. During embryogenesis, some of the mesenchyme cells differentiate into chondroblasts, which then further differentiate and later become chondrocytes. The chondrocytes are responsible for the secretion of the cartilage matrix, which is composed of Type II collagen fibrils suspended in a concentrated solution of proteoglycans (Hukins 1984). The proteoglycans in cartilage consist of both chondroitin sulfate and keratan sulfate.

Analysis of the composition of cartilage reveals that approximately 10 percent of the tissue's volume consists of chondrocytes, anywhere from 10 to 30 percent consists of the collagen fibers, 3 to 10 percent are proteoglycans and the rest of the volume is made up of water, inorganic salts, lipids, glycoproteins and other matrix proteins (Hukins 1984). Microscopically, the collagen content of articular cartilage varies from layer to layer, as do the chondrocytes' patterns. In both cases the superficial layer reveals a more compact alignment of fibers and cells that are parallel to the articular surface. The tissue in the middle zone is sparsely and randomly distributed. This possibly accounts for the concentration of proteoglycans and water. The deep-zone tissue forms radically oriented columns with the collagen fibers that actually anchor to the underlying bone. The chondrocytes provide the border between calcified and non-calcified tissue (Hukins 1984).

We have already reviewed some of the functional properties of cartilage. Specifically, cartilage is specialized dense connective tissue that is able to deform under pressure, recover its original shape after that pressure is removed, and support various skeletal junctions (Frankel 1980). Cartilage is avascular: the chondrocytes within the matrix actually secrete a chemical that inhibits the formation of blood vessels. Accordingly, all cellular activities, e.g., waste removal and nourishment, occur via diffusion (Lowen 1990). In

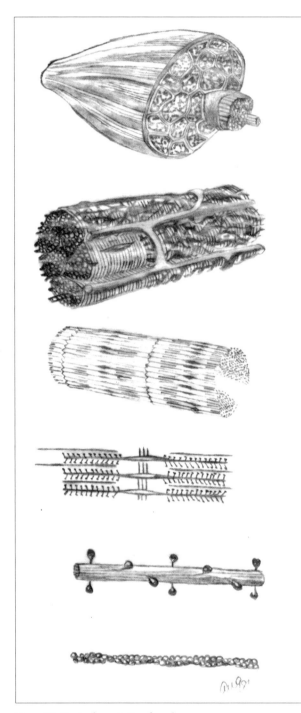

Figure 11. Structural organization of muscle.

addition to being without blood vessels, the cartilage is also without a nerve supply.

Hyaline, elastic, and articular cartilage are all classified according to the abundance collagen fibers and their proteoglycan content. Hyaline cartilage is the most common of all the types. It covers the articular surface of bones, supports the *tracheal tubes* and the *larynx* of the respiratory tract, and connects the ribs to the *sternum*. Because of its high proportion of elastic fibers, elastin cartilage is different from hyaline cartilage, although it consists of similar collagen fiber (Type II). These elastin fibers add resiliency and flexibility to the tissue. Elastin cartilage is found in the outer ear, epiglottis, and tip of the nose.

The third type of cartilage is called *fibrocartilage* and represents a composite of hyaline cartilage and fibrous connective tissue. There is very little ground substance and a high proportion of collagen fibers (Type I) in fibrocartilage. Its density helps create an extremely durable tissue. It is found in the *meniscus* of joints, *annulus fibrosis* of the intervertebral disc, within the attachments of tendons to bones and between the bones of the pelvis. The tissue resists compression, absorbs and distributes shock, and prevents damage from bone to bone contact (Lowen 1990).

Bone and cartilage are supportive connective tissues that help distribute high amounts of stress and strain throughout the body's framework, as is evidenced by the positional nature of the skeleton and the organization of transitional tissues at their articulations.

Muscle

While the collagen content of bone and cartilage permits remarkable compensatory properties within those tissues, its presentation as loose and dense connective tissue in muscle allows for tremendous functional capabilities. There are three types of muscle found in the body—smooth, skeletal, and cardiac—but this discussion will focus only on the skeletal.

Skeletal muscle accounts for over 40 percent

of the total body weight in the average person. The connective tissue within this plays an integral role in the performance of many functions, including static and dynamic posture, support, movement, and maintenance of body temperature. Muscle's connective tissue helps create a structure that has properties similar to both connective tissue proper and bone. Bone has a combination of solid material in the form of the calcium salts, flexible materials in the form of collagen, and an organic matrix that yields a tissue that is ingeniously supportive in regards to structure, yet flexible enough to allow for significant bending, shearing, rotation, compression, distraction and torquing. The connective tissue of the muscle's functional unit, the *myofibril,* plays an equally important part in structural organization. (See Figure 11.)

The muscle fibers range from 10 to 100 mn and are 1 to 3 cm in length (Hukins 1984). Connective tissue helps compartmentalize and separate each successive layer within the muscle fiber, and also allows for communication and transport, among other functions.

The deepest layer of connective tissue, the *endomysium,* is a loose connective tissue, and it directly encompasses each muscle fiber while connecting it to adjacent muscle fibers. These bundles of fibers are called *fascicles.* Each fascicle is enclosed in a dense connective tissue sheath called the *perimysium.* The perimysium surrounds bundles of fascicles, just as the endomysium surrounds the individual muscle fibers. Another dense connective tissue that surrounds these bundles of fascicles is called the *epimysium.* This tissue not only surrounds the muscle; it has additional connective tissue fibers that attach to its surrounding structures (Fitton-Jackson 1965).

Within the layer of endomysium there are *satellite cells* that functionduring damage repair of the muscle fiber. The perimysium and epimysium house the nerves and vasculature for the muscle fiber (Lowen 1990). The epimysium and the perimysium continue beyond each end of the muscle fibers and band together to form a tendon that then blends with the periosteum of the bone at its attachment. The attachment, evident under a microscope, reveals gradations of tissues referred to as *transitional zones.* The zones have characteristic delineations and are differentiated in the following manner: Zone 1: collagen fibers; Zone 2: *unmineralized fibrocartilage;* Zone 3: *mineralized fibrocartilage;* and Zone 4: *cortical bone.*

The tonus of the muscle unit ranges from complete flaccidity (during pathologic or surgical states) to being extremely rigid and hard, as occurs with maximum contraction. This capability of shifting from a sol (solution) to a gel state is a characteristic of connective tissue and its ground substance that is universal throughout the body. Juhan refers to this property as a liquid crystal (Schoitz 1958). Variations of this trait are based on location, function, stress, and strain.

Tendons have a unique arrangement of structures based on regional needs. (See Figure 8.) Loose areolar connective tissue surrounds the tendon and is call the *paratenon.* This material forms a sheath that enhances gliding while adding protection for the tendon. When tendons are exposed to increased levels of friction, for instance at the wrist joint, an additional layer of protection can be found underneath the paratenon. This is referred to as the *epitenon.* It is capable of producing *synovial fluid* via synovial cells, which help further facilitate the gliding of the tissues (Nortrop 1952). There are bundles of fibers that are held together by *endotenon,* which is synonymous with the epimysium and perimysium, from the muscle unit.

Dense Irregular and Regular Connective Tissue

In dense irregular connective tissue, the collagen fibers are arranged in a manner that lets them withstand stress from all directions. It is found in joint capsules, soft tissue capsules around organs such as the spleen, liver, and kidneys, and in the periosteum and aponeuroses (Cantu and Grodin 1992). The multi-directional capability of this tissue to provide support, protection, and strength makes it a unique structure and difficult to replace once it is injured.

Examples of dense regular connective tissue include aponeuroses and elastic tissue. Aponeuroses help attach muscle to other structures, while elastic tissue provides resiliency to a structure allowing it to stretch. Dense irregular tissue is found in the larynx and respiratory pathways as well as in blood vessels.

Alveolar Tissue

As the ratio of collagen to ground substance shifts to favor ground substance, connective tissue is referred to as loose connective tissue or areolar tissue. Along with the ground substance, which is loose connective tissue's predominate component, this areolar tissue is suited to absorbing significant shocks without sustaining perceptible injury. There are elastic fibers in this tissue that give resiliency as well as the ability to move in any direction. This tissue also creates a functional space between the subdermis and underlying muscle. This component allows the muscle to contract without disturbing the tissue above; conversely any external force on the skin does not encroach on the underlying muscle, for example, pinching. The elastic fibers allow for the stretching of the loose connective tissue. This layer also has a close association with the *circulatory system;* the intake and outgo of essential nutrients, carbon dioxide, oxygen, and waste products occur as an ongoing process (Lowen 1990). This tissue is also found in the superficial and deep fascial layers, as well as around nerve sheaths.

No tissue in the body, whether it is connective tissue, muscle, nerve, or epithelium exists in isolation. All of these tissues act upon and are acted upon by other physical, chemical, energetic entities, which together comprise a network of more organized structures we classify as systems. All systems are interactive and integrated within, among, and between many levels. System designations such as the allopathic profession has delineated are merely subdivisions of organizational frameworks. The subdivisions perform a seemingly cohesive and linear function or fall within a group of homogenous tissues that have been labeled according to that function. Overlap between the systems is inherent to our body's framework and function. This overlapping of many systems reflects the importance of the continuity and contiguity of the connective tissue.

PART TWO

CONNECTIVE TISSUE DYSFUNCTION

CHAPTER 10

THE HISTOPATHOLOGY OF CONNECTIVE TISSUE AND THE STAGES OF HEALING

The reactions of connective tissue to various external and internal stimuli have been examined and outlined by many researchers (Cantu and Grodin 1992; Bourdillion 1970; Lowen 1990). There exists a core mechanism within the tissue that reacts uniformly to a loss of homeostasis, no matter what the causes or how many different systems are involved. The entire process has been divided into two, three, or four stages of healing by various writers (Cantu and Grodin 1992; Weiss; Lowen 1990). This discussion will include three stages, outlined as follows: (1) *Inflammation stage*; (2) *fibroplastic stage*; and (3) *remodeling/maturation stage*. (See Figure 12.)

Inflammation occurs immediately after a trauma in response to the destruction or irritation of vascularized tissues. The specialized cells needed at this time of healing generally come from the vascular tissue. Protein messengers called "mediators" control the specialized cells. Over 300 cell-synthesized mediators have been identified, as we noted earlier.

Four Stages of Tissue Healing

Necrosis (tissue degeneration) occurs secondary to *lysosomal enzyme release* within minutes after an initial trauma. Via *autolysis*, the damaged cells are eliminated along with any surrounding tissue debris. The blood vessels that have been severed at the time of the injury allow blood to pour into the wound, coagulating and sealing the vessels and creating a *hematoma*. The arteries, veins, and lymphatic vessels are sealed quickly after the injury, creating a *vasoconstriction* that lasts only momentarily, before reflex *vasodilatation* increases blood flow and causes swelling.

Concurrent with the vascular response to injury, other mediators function as a result of clot-

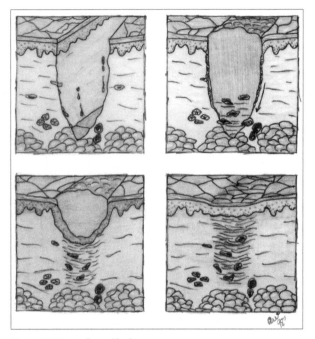

Figure 12. Stages of wound healing.

ting factor XII. *Capillary permeability* and *edema* increase secondary to bradykinin release; *fibrinolysis* counteracts clot formation; the *phagocytosis* of damaged tissue ensues; and *coagulation* to reduce blood loss continues (Weiss 1984). The phagocytosis prepares the wound for repair or regeneration while also helping to prevent infection.

Other responses to trauma that occur almost at the time of injury include the stimulation of mast cells and basophilic secretion of histamine and heparin. Both of these substances stimulate local neurons for a *withdrawal response*, while histamine works additionally with serotonin to increase vascular permeability by relaxing smooth muscle and vascular tissues in the vessel walls. With the increased blood flow, there is an acceleration of the flow of nutrients into the area and an increase in the removal of waste products and toxins.

White blood cells (leukocytes) migrate to the trauma site, partially because of changes in the electrostatic charges near the injury. Once there, these leukocytes are responsible for increased vascular permeability and the release of leukotriene, prostaglandin, and *platelet activating factor*. The leukocytes further release *hydrolytic enzymes,* which lead to *archidonic acid* production. The release of additional polypeptide proteins adds to the prolonged increase in tissue permeability (Weiss 1984).

Tissue clean up is aided further by monocytes, *microcytes*, microphages and free macrophages, as well as fixed macrophages. Free macrophages, derived from the monocytes in the blood, migrate toward the injury site and squeeze through the endothelial cells by the process of diapedesis. The macrophage is also very sensitive to chemicals released by cells at the injury site. This process of attraction is called "chemotaxis" (Fitton-Jackson 1965) as we noted before. Plasma cells also use a chemical approach via antibody production to help clean up tissues after injury.

Inflammation is necessary if healing is to occur. If there is too little inflammation, healing will be slowed; conversely, if there is too much inflammation, scarring can be excessive. Inflammatory responses are not necessarily reflective of actual tissue damage. For example, a minor impact to a bursa may cause significant edema with only minor soft tissue damage. A fractured bone at times yields minimal edema. Hardy notes that the macrophage is the key factor in regulating the inflammatory response—especially its role in fibroblast recruitment and scar production (DeLaporte and Siegfried 1983).

Phagocytosis is an integral component in wound healing. Equally important is the *neurovascularization* of the traumatized area. This latter process is called *angiogenesis*. It occurs when the *arterioles* and *venuoles* combine to form a new capillary loop. When this occurs, *fibrinolysin* helps dissolve *fibrin plugs* within the blood and lymph vessels, which subsequently help reduce localized edema. The inflammation phase can last from several minutes to several days. (See Figure 13.)

Tissues can undergo two types of mechanisms when progressing from the inflammatory stage to the fibroplastic stage: regeneration and repair. (See Figures 13 and 14.) True regeneration occurs when the new lattices are identical in both function and structure to the tissue they are replacing. During repair, the new tissues are not identical to the original matrix in structure or function. The best example of tissue regeneration is bone healing. Tissue repair includes any reorganization that involves scarring. Depending on the source and location of inflammation, certain conditions arise where the body may want to immobilize the tissue in order to inhibit further movement. This will be discussed later in "Adhesions, Fibrosis, and Atrophy," Chapter 11.

The second phase of tissue repair can start two days after the initial injuryand continue for more than two months. This is referred to as the *fibroplastic stage of healing*, so named because of the dominance of the fibroplastic activity. This stage can actually start before the completion of phagocytosis. Concurrent with the revascularization and fibroblast proliferation, macrophage and hystiocyte activity make way for the appearance of granulation tissue. This tissue appears approximately four days after the injury and is typically Type III collagen. Type III collagen usually has a weak electrostatic charge and bonds in an unstable manner with other fibers. As maturation progresses, the Type III tissue is replaced by Type I tissue, which has stronger cross linking and covalent bondings (Hukins 1984).

Prior to the laying down of a fibroplastic network and in order to initiate repair and regeneration, the actual closure of the wound is achieved. Plasma and blood proteins form a clot. This encloses the inflamed region and inhibits the spread of cellular debris and infection. The epithelial tissue closest to the injury site regenerates identical cells, which marginalize the wound. These cells, along with myofibroblast cells, ultimately shrink and close the wound. Further digestive enzymes help mobilize non-viable tissue from the wound such as *eschar*. As fibroblast activity increases, the demand for increased vascularization also rises in order to meet the metabolic need of the tissue (DeLaporte and Siegfried 1983). A key aspect of the fibroplastic stage of healing has to do with the fibroblast. Since the exudates that contain the fibroblast migrate throughout the entire injury site, the new collagen fibrous network is extensive. Fibroblasts secrete *procollagen,* which, when cleaved, become *tropocollagen,* the basic unit of the collagen fiber. Initial activity brings Type III collagen, which is characterized by weak hydrostatic bonding, to the repair site, where there are smaller fibrils and fewer cross-links. If the tissue remains as it is deposited, long-term structural weakness of the area can be expected. In most cases the Type III collagen is replaced by Type I collagen that is characterized by co- and trivalent bonding. This means that there are stronger cross-links for a larger number of fibrils.

Another aspect of *fibroblast synthesis* is the production of the ground substance and proteoglycan aggregates that contain glycosaminoglycans (GAGs) and hyaluronic acid. The ground substance has been likened to a huge electrostatic sponge, which in turn binds with water and helps maintain critical interfiber distance during scar maturation. For the manual practitioner, this cross-linking allows for early controlled mobilization without potential damage and recurrence of the repair cycle. (DeLaporte 1983.)

The last stage of tissue repair is called the maturation or remodeling phase (See Figure 16.) Each tissue in the body has a different capability for repair/regeneration. For example, cartilage and ligaments heal slowly, secondary to the decreased number of local specialized cells available for the repair process. Bone and muscle heal relatively rapidly because of the large number of readily available reparation cells (Weiss 1984). Yet a

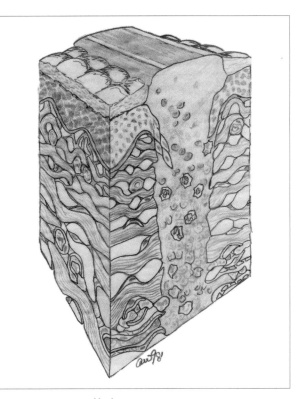

Figure 13. Stage 1 wound healing.

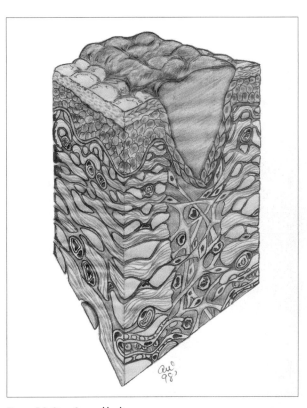

Figure 14. Stage 2 wound healing.

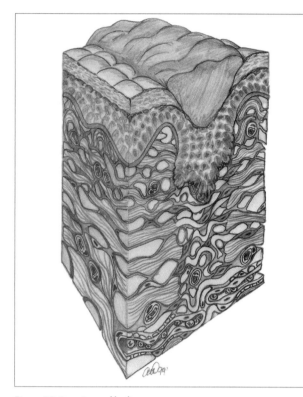

Figure 15. Stage 3 wound healing.

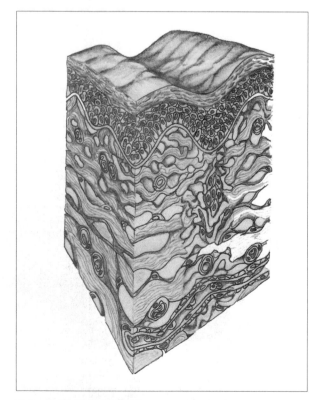

Figure 16. Stages of wound healing.

structure's ability to begin the repair process does not reflect how well it can regenerate. Although muscle and tendon heal rapidly, their sequelae yield only scar tissue, which structurally is not as stable as the original matrix of the core tissue. The younger an individual happens to be, typically the better the regenerative/reparative process. Recent clinical research is showing some significant gains in the reparative processes of cardiac and neural tissue (Barral 1988; Lowen 1996; Lowen 1992).

As well as stronger cross-linking between collagenous fibrils and the restoration of ground substance, this last stage is marked by decreased cellular activity. The actual cell production slowly increases, with a more normal biomechanical balance and a focus on homeostasis. Part of the remaining cellular activity includes collagen synthesis, which proceeds at a high rate during remodeling. Under normal conditions no increase in scar mass occurs (DeLaporte 1983). During this last stage, *collagenase* balance between catabolic (lysis) and anabolic (synthesis) factors is maintained. Collagenase is an integral enzyme, which is capable of cleaving the strong cross-link in tropocollagen molecules. An imbalance in this process, such as *lysis inhibition,* which can occur secondary to *hypoxia,* can lead to excessive scarring (hypertrophic) and *reloids.* This can also be responsible for progressive *fibrosis,* which can affect tissues uninvolved in the original trauma. Manual practitioners who treat burns have recognized that direct pressure on scars creates a pseudo-anoxic state that stimulates lysis progression (DeLaporte and Siegfried 1983).

There are two theories relating to tissue healing. The first is the *induction theory,* which simply states that a scar attempts to mimic, via synthesis and lysis, the characteristics of the tissue that is healing. The second is the *tension theory,* which refers to internal and external stresses that directly and indirectly affect the organization of the collagen framework.

Examples of the forces that can act on the tissue include passive range of motion, active range of motion, temperature changes, splinting, fascial tension (including 3-planar myofascial fulcrums), muscle tension, and joint mobilization (including hard, soft, and partial soft joint). When comparing types of stretching, it has been noted that short, sustained stretching affects the elastic components of connective tissue more than other types of stretching does. Other forms of stretching yield only a temporary change in tissue length; low load, long duration stresses have more of an affect on the plastic component of the connective tissue (Cantu and Grodin 1992).

Clinically, the general shift towards early onset mobilization has become more the rule than the exception. Traditionally, the focus of rehabilitation was placed on the collagenous component of connective tissue, with only peripheral attention to the ground substance as an indirect factor in tissue mobilization. We ourselves view the ground substance as being at least as important in the healing process, if not more important, than the collagen/elastin components of connective tissue.

The maturation component of wound healing represents a logical extension of the remodeling phase. This phase is quite variable in duration, depending on the tissue involved and the requirements for restoration of normal movement at the injured site. Ligamentous healing, for instance, continues well beyond a year's time at the microscopic level; yet within six to eight weeks of an injury, most of these tissues can withstand some weight bearing and mobilization.

CHAPTER 11

ADHESIONS, FIBROSIS, AND ATROPHY

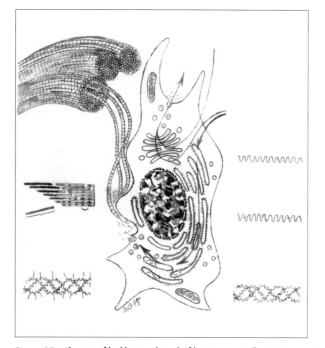

Figure 17a. The active fibroblast regulates the fibrotic process (adhesion) involving the collagen fibers,

Adhesions and Fixations

Adhesions and *fixations* are specific classifications pertinent to the scarring process. (See Figures 17a and 17b.) Adhesions or fixations occur secondary to the normal healing process. Exudates occur in areas of irritation from trauma, eventually thickening in order to eliminate motion at the particular site. Without the introduction of controlled movement and a rehydration of the spaces in between the new collagen tissues with GAGs, proteoglycans and hyaluronic acid, the adhesion/fixation creates a whole new axis of motion that perpetuates a point of continued irritation and creates new restrictions on motion. In *hard joints,* for example the *glenohumeral joint,* these restrictions can at times be manipulated manually, as long as the force does not create greater problems after manipulation. Often this type of soft tissue restriction is surgically addressed; but in many cases this creates more adhesions. Barral notes that the aggressive manipulation of soft tissue adhesions or fixations can actually irritate the uninvolved tissue that surrounds the stronger restriction, thus creating more tenacious scarring (Barral 1993).

Secondary to an adhesion, a continuous state of mechanical irritation can affect many systems that are far removed from the involved site. Under nonpathologic conditions, the normal motion and activities of daily living maintain the movement potential of tissues along an established axis of motion. A new scar can easily shift one or more of the normal axes of motion in either soft or hard tissues. This creates a source of irritation that perpetuates the scarring process and the chronic pain cycle, and causes further loss of biomechanical balance (Lowen 1996).

Fibrosis

Fibrosis, as a process, is less linear than scarring, which typically occurs step by step in sequence. Fibrosis usually involves the connective tissues and structures of an entire region. Cantu and Grodin note that fibrosis has none of the lines of demarcation that are the attributes of scarring (Cantus and Grodin 1992). The process of fibrosis can occur in at least two distinct fashions. The first may be associated with the synthesis/lysis imbalance of collagen production from a nearby traumatic site. Studies have indicated that the process of fibrosis is accelerated during wound repair, and that neighboring tissue can become involved. We ourselves have noticed fibrosis to occur along lengthy kinematic chains, e.g., cranium to sacrum, as well as progressively through tissue distant from the traumatized area. In one case, an apparently simple palmer restriction created during surgery for a trigger finger, progressively fibrosed tissue through the *volar mid forearm.*

(Weiselfish) Giammatteo has found that since "head-on" type head injuries generally result in a condition known as *descended sacrum,* there is a high correlation between such injuries and *fibrosis of the spinal cord.* She found that the altered biomechanics created a sustained pull on the *dural tube* secondary to the *caudal displacement of the sacrum,* and that this apparently predisposed the tissue and lead to fibrosis (Lowen and Weiselfish 1996).

The concept of spinal fibrosis was discussed by Dr. DeLaporte et al. in 1983. Neurosurgeons discovered that *spinal arachnoiditis* can actually develop into *spinal fibrosis.* The etiology can be from surgery, epidermal injections, myelograms, and other causes. Its evolution is unpredictable although self-limiting. Dr. DeLaporte stated that spinal fibrosis comprises several syndromes, all based on the same anatomical substrate. He examined extended adherences between the elements of *cauda equina,* with thickening and *induration of the meninges,* frequently accompanied by the

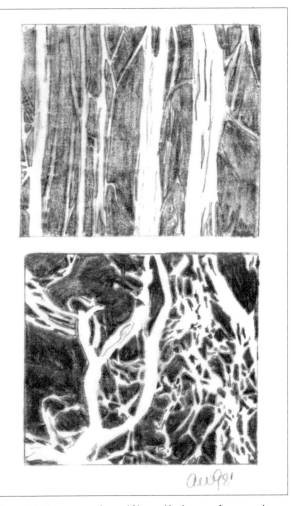

Figure 17b. Arrangement of normal fibers and healing scar after two weeks.

formation of cysts and the obliteration of the *sub-dural space* (Akeson, Woo, Amiel, et al. 1973). On a microscopic level he found a progression of pathologic changes which he described in three phases: (1) an inflammation of *pia-arachnoid membrane* with *hyperemia* and thickening of the roots of the *cauda equina;* (2) progression of fibroplatsic proliferation and deposition of collagen as well as a diminution of thickening of the roots and adherence between themselves and pia-arachnoid membrane; and (3) the completion of an autoimmune inflammatory process, with complete encapsulation of the hyperemic and atrophied nerve roots with marked proliferation to the pia-arachnoid tissues and dense deposition of collagen. He goes into several theories as possible explanations of spinal fibrosis (DeLaporte and Siegfried 1983). Brieg extensively reviews the concept of spinal cord fibrosis in his research (Akeson and Amiel 1967).

Cell Atrophy

Cell atrophy is yet another condition where connective tissue can be altered negatively, creating an avenue for potential injury. Secondary to stress response, metabolic activities can decrease or cease altogether. Once started in this cycle, e.g., from immobilization, energy production decreases along with other functions. This leads to degeneration and increased vulnerability to injury. The effect of immobility on the ground substance as well as on collagen and collagen production will be discussed in conjunction with nontraumatic reaction of connective tissue (Weiss 1984).

Connective Tissue and Immobilization

One of the many frustrations encountered by rehabilitation practitioners on an almost daily basis is the soft tissue sequelae that result from *immobilization.* Immobilization occurs in both static and dynamic situations. The typical type of immobilization most practitioners experience is a static form that involves braces, casts, wraps,

traction, fusion, etc. Other immobilizations that occur are those secondary to minor traumas, which can lead to protective muscle spasm or infections, and further lead to adhesions. Still another from of immobilization could be classified as progressive in nature, such as bone spurring in osteoarthritis, or the immobility noted secondary to fibromyalgia. At some level, with all these examples, there exists a condition where either internal or external fixation of body parts occurs Akeson and Amiel (Akeson and Amiel et al. 1973) noted the importance of mechanical forces for tissue homeostasis, and how little research has been performed dealing with the inter- and intracellular adaptation of localized tissue responses, based on structure and function. In the absence of stress, the rapid deterioration of muscle and connective tissue, i.e., cartilage, tendons, ligaments, synovial joints and capsules, is imminent. Most practitioners agree that the rate of atrophy is much higher than the rate of *hypertrophy* of the same tissues. Therapists have been obliged in their early treatment to concentrate on mobilization instead of rest. It has been noted that, at least at times, atrophy is far more detrimental to the remobilization of tissues than scarring (DeLaporte and Siegfried 1983). A core concept of immobilization can be drawn from a correlative application of *Wolff's law* which states that tissues adapt to the stresses applied or not applied to them.

Significant research on immobilization has been preformed, much of it on animals (Donatelli and Owens-Burkhardt 1981), extrapolated to fit human anatomy and function. Much of the research has been performed on nontraumatized joints, or surgically induced traumatic joints and soft tissues. Where possible, these delineations will be highlighted.

Biochemical and biomechanical responses to immobilization appear consistent in the research. Fibrofatty connective tissue proliferation was found within the joint spaces of rabbit and rat knees after fifteen days of immobilization (Weiss;

Noyes 1977). The entire joint capsule, including articulating and nonarticulating surfaces, were exposed to the connective tissue blanket which eventually caused a loss of the whole joint space via adhesions and mature scar (Donatelli and Owens-Burkhardt 1981; Baker, Thomas, and Kirkaldy-Willis 1968; Trais 1961). Similar histological changes have been noted in other rabbit, dog, rat, human, and primate studies (DeLaporte and Siegfried 1983). Knee and facet joints have been examined in humans (DeLaporte and Siegfried 1983). The aforementioned *periarticular* and *synovial tissue* changes have some similarities to articular cartilage secondary to immobilization. The nonarticulating surfaces of the studied joints incur changes secondary to the proliferating fibrofatty connective tissue. The articulating surfaces were covered completely with tissue within thirty days (Trais 1961). Among other changes noted were a thinning of the articular cartilage, fibrillation, and loss of matrix staining, distortion, and shrinking of chondrocytes (Parker and Keefer 1935).

Additionally, cartilage is subject to the sequelae of compression or immobilization due to adhesions. Salter and Field noted pressure necrosis as early as six days postimmobilization in a compromised position of continued pressure. Ulceration of the cartilage with erosion to *subchondral bone* is possible as well as fibrillation, necrosis, and cellular distortion (Lanier). In lesions where articular cartilage damage was confined to the superficial layers, regeneration was possible secondary to the remaining chondrocytes in the deeper layer (Salter and Field 1960). In cases where damage was to and through the deeper layer, the surfaces were invaded by primative mesenchymal tissue (Parker and Keefer 1935). Other components studied by researchers dealt with the amount of immobilization (total/partial) suffered during treatment. Whether it was partial or total, within forty-five to ninety days the joints were found to be essentially rigid.

Important research regarding constant versus intermittent pressures on bone and connective tissue has helped shift our rehabilitation focus from rest to motion. Trias performed an experiment in which he applied four hours of compression each day to an immobilized knee joint: he found no signs of degenerative changes (Salter and Field 1960). Woo immobilized rabbit knees with casts for one to sixteen weeks without compression. Remobilization lasted no longer than the period of immobilization. Reexamination of the articular surfaces revealed decreased thickness and decreased staining of the intercellular ground substance with some cellular abnormalities, but the overall evidence showed that sequelae from immobilization could be reversed (Evans, Eggers, et al. 1960). In Evans' 1960 study, remobilization was accomplished through abrupt forced movement, active range of motion, and passive range of motion within the available range. Within an approximate thirty-day window, range of motion could be regained even though major cartilage deficits appeared nonreversible. Beyond thirty days, the knee joint did not regain full functional movement (Trais 1961). Conversely, researchers noted irreversible damage to tissue during remobilization of rabbits that were allowed to exercise freely.

Enwemeka (Enwemeka 1991), in his study of tendons, found that immobilization of three or more weeks induced progressive disorganization of collagen and a decrease in the size of the collagen fibrils. Muscle lengthening produced a temporary reversal of this atrophy. He went on to further study the effects of the early loading of tissues with mechanical stress. Because atrophy is marked within days of tendon repair and immobilization, remobilization was initiated passively and as early as possible. Not only did he find mobility improved with passive range of motion, but strength gains were noted as well (Hardy 1989).

Muscle atrophy occurs rapidly, i.e., 50 percent of the total loss occurs within the first week of immobilization, due to a decrease in protein synthesis leading to a great loss of muscle protein. This process starts within hours of the immobilization and can be minimized by functional loading of the joint and passive mobilization. McDonough reviewed two different studies that examined the effects of exercise on articular cartilage (Salter, Bell, and Kelley 1981). In a 1950 study, Saaf showed that the number of cells per unit volume initially increased with three weeks exercise but then decreased after that time. Lanier concluded one to six hours of exercise on a treadmill did not contribute to joint degeneration in mice. Ekholm and Norback found histological changes in articular cartilage in rabbits after exercise when compared to nonexercised limbs. The cells were representative of degenerative changes. It was suggested that stress deprivation from the loss of joint movement may cause degeneration changes secondary to decreased nutritional availability. In other words, exercise performed too early or too vigorously can lead to deterioration of tissues, and biological recovery can lag behind functional return. This is in keeping with the present authors' experience that *structure dictates function and that function influences structure,* especially at the microscopic level.

A popular treatment regimen *(continuous passive range of motion)* has evolved from the extensive research on articular cartilage immobilization and remobilization. Continuous passive range of motion has been found to have significant beneficial effects on connective tissue. Among these effects are: improved removal of blood from the postsurgical joint; a reduction in articular cartilage damage in septic arthritis and improved rate; and improved quality of repair of tendon, bone, ligament, and cartilage.

Microscopic Changes Secondary to Immobilization

Other tissue component alterations due to immobilization occur at the microscopic molecular level. Histochemical changes in the connective tissue concurrent with immobilization can be observed in several components of the matrix. A loss of glycosaminoglycans (GAGs) is the most prominent component of immobilization of tissues; specifically, chondroitin-4, chondroitin sulfate-6, hyaluronic acid, and at a lesser level, dermatan sulfate. The concentration of loss ranges from 30 percent to approximately 40 percent (Donatelli and Owens-Burkhardt 1981). The proteoglycan monomer aggregates, consisting of the GAGs and hyaluronic acid, correspondingly lose water. Water content loss in connective tissue ranges from 65 to 70 percent in the extracellular fluid. The extensive need for water as a lubricant in connective tissue has been well established. Because the half-life of collagen is between 300 and 500 days and the half-life of GAGs is between approximately two and seven days, the lubricating effect from the tissue's water binding capacity plays an even greater role in generation (Gamble; Edwards; Max 1984).

Other factors lead to further tissue degradation. As the amount of GAG's and hyaluronic acid decreases, the critical fiber distance needed between collagen fibers is compromised. This can lead to excessive cross-linking and adhesions and fixation. Gamble suggests that *lysosomal hydrolyses* are responsible for GAG degradation, while Akeson and Amiel et al. feel it is a reduction of hyaluronic acid synthesis secondary to immobilization that is responsible for GAG and water loss (Donatelli and Owens-Burkhard 1981). This is facilitated by a homeostatic feedback loop based on physical forces within the connective tissue ground substance. Not only does a fibril to fibril fixation occur with a decrease in the fluid volume of the ground substance, but the needed stresses provide a balance mechanism for any newly synthesized collagen. Without the pressure, new tissue is laid down in a random manner. The viscoealstic properties become compromised as there is a shift from sol (solution) to gel, and a degenerative cycle leads to clinical symptoms of joint stiffness, loss of motion, and ultimately pathology.

Very little attention has been focused on this

reflex mechanical loop of communication between cell and system. Hemler described cell membrane receptors called *integrins* that may be responsible for this phenomena (Hemler 1987). Dahners (Dahners 1986) characterized the glycoproteins as having a primary role with collagen, laminin and fibronectin. Fibronectin is associated with inter- and extracellular matrixes, cell migration, and the reticuloendothelial system, which ultimately has been shown to facilitate wound healing.

Collagen loss secondary to immobilization occurs slowly. Within the first nine weeks there is a loss of 5 to 50 percent; by the twelfth week, collagen mass loss has been recorded at 29 percent. Akeson and Ameiel and Woo noted that since collagen degradation and turnover is higher than its synthesis, contractures are unlikely to be a product of the latter (Evans, Eggers, et al. 1960.)

External immobilization can obviously lead to internal immobilization in the presence of an inflammatory process or a loss of the mechanoreceptor type reflex loop in the connective tissues. Secondary to a loss of required and necessary stress on structures, this reflex loop initiates a degeneration cycle that is marked by a significant loss of GAGs and water. Without these essential elements, the *critical fiber distance* between collagen fibers is lost, and this leads to an increase in cross-linking and eventually scarring and adhesions. The rehabilitation expert must be aware of this process as it occurs, and under what conditions. The inflammatory process will entail extra wound/trauma healing sequelae that need to be addressed early in the rehabilitation phase.

Restoration of Movement

The restoration of movement in all aspects of immobilization is quite essential for rehabilitation. Internal fixation occurs secondary to infections, malposture, overuse syndromes, etc. It causes adhesions, scarring, and fibrosis, and can be initiated by traumatic exudates. When movement potential is assessed, all articulations must be considered joints. No joint is so small that it can be disregarded. In fact, we observe that the joints that present with the greatest potential for dysfunction are the smallest ones such as the sacroiliac joint, cranial joints, accessory joints, vertebral body/endplate joints, the *chondrosternal* and *chondrocostal* joint, interarticular spaces, lumbosacral joints, occipitoatlantal and soft tissue joints.

Progressive immobilization from disease processes requires special attention by the therapist in regard to understanding etiology, outcomes, and potential interventions. For example, a process such as fibromyalgia needs to be examined on a system-by-system basis. The constructs of the connective tissue system involved in this pathology interact inclusively as well as exclusively with no less than the circulatory, lymphatic, neurologic, skeletal, craniosacral, visceral, endocrine, muscular, integumentary and reticuloendothelial systems. In general, all of these "joints" and systems need evaluation. Assessment and intervention can be tissue specific. In the situation of the muscular system's relationship to connective tissue, protective muscle spasm is often a by-product of this process. The physiologic effect is an excessive, high-frequency discharge relayed via the *primary afferents*. This leads to excessive *efferent (alpha) outflow,* coupled with an increase in *gamma activity* and *muscle spindle hyperactivity.* A *facilitated spinal segment* is a potential outcome. The resulting sustained *protective muscle spasm* can affect local tissue drainage within the lymphatics by altering interstitial pressure levels. Without appropriate movement of waste products from the interstitium to the venous capillaries and especially to the lymphatic channels, the ground substance eventually changes from sol (solution) to gel. At the very least, there is a significant irritation of the free nerve endings in the interstitial tissues. Pathologies left untreated perpetuate global physiologic, metabolic, and mechanical changes far removed from the symptomatic areas.

Trigger Points and Tender Points

Trigger Points à la Janet Travell, M.D.

Definition: A trigger point is a focus of hyperirritability in a tissue that, when compressed, is locally tender and, if sufficiently hypersensitive, gives rise to referred pain, and sometimes to referred autonomic phenomena and proprioceptive distortion. Types include: myofascial, cutaneous, fascial, ligamentous, and periosteal trigger points.

Tender Points à la Lawrence Jones, D.O.

"These tense, tender and edematous spots...are located in the deeper tissue of the muscles, tendons, ligaments, and fascia and occasionally the joint line or suture. They measure 1 cm across (or less) with the most acute point about 3 mm in diameter. There may be multiple tender points for one specific joint dysfunction or they may extend for a few centimeters along a muscle, or may be arranged in a chain. The patient is usually unaware of the tender point's presence until it is palpated. Tender points in the extremities are often found in a painless area opposite to the site of pain and apparent weakness." (Leach 1986). (See Table IV.)

Drs. Travell and Simons' texts on myofascial pain and dysfunction (Travell and Simons 1983) elaborately map out the musculoskeletal origins of the condition revealed in muscle biopsy where, with manipulation of the contractile tissue or superficial fascia, a reproducible *referred pain pattern* was created (Jones 1991). Trigger points are typically not synonymous with acupuncture points, motor points, skin or scar tissue points, Chapman's Reflexes or tender points (Leach 1986; Jones 1991). All these points have similar locations to trigger points (areas or zones) but are not identical to them.

Understanding the significance of "the points" in both the Travell and Jones modalities is essential for utilizing their subsequent methods of treatment. Travell's Trigger Points elicit a specific pain pattern. Recognition of the reference zone associated with each muscle is a keystone for complete diagnosis. Even though the referred pain patterns are reproducible and predictable, confusion arises when, as is often the case, more than one point is involved. A practitioner must recognize when patterns overlap, as well as the level of severity which exists, in order to gain the best possible advantage for treatment.

Jones' Tender Point patterns as trigger point reference zones are consistent with Travell, yet many of Jones' points are located in a site completely opposite of where a pain complaint is noted. For instance, many patients who complain of low back pain in the region of the fifth lumbar vertebra (L5) and the first sacral vertebra (S1) experience tenderness in the corresponding anterior tender points in several structures including the area of the ilium and pubic bones. All of the anterior points are typically exquisitely tender, although the patient's original complaint is of posterior pain. From a subjective viewpoint, it may not appear obvious why a referred pain pattern is so far removed from the area of complaint. The hypothetical physiologic core of the dysfunction, (protective muscle spasm) provides an explanation (Leach 1986; Korr and Wright 1947).

Diagnoses

There are many diagnostic terms that in themselves imply the impact of fascia on pathology. Some of these terms are becoming more accepted in allopathic medicine; others are already being overutilized as "catch basin" terms to include any subcategories of similar findings. Such diagnostic terms include: *fibrositis, myofibrosities, fibromyositis, intestinal myofibrosities, fibromyalgia, rheumatic myalgia, myalgiac spots, panniculosis or panniculitis, idiopathic myalgia, muscular rheumatism, chronic fatigue syndrome,* and *fibrositic spots.* Many of these classifications are different names for the same clinical finding. The authors present these as *connective tissue syndromes.* Categorizing signs and symptoms, especially in a system, continues to be a pitfall in allopathic medicine. Once they have identified the relevant categories, practitioners tend to limit their research and subsequent thinking when looking for additional causative factors. Too often, linear thinking in regards to the human body besets the crucial need for non-linear approaches to the interpretation of somatic dysfunction.

Table IV

	Travell Trigger Points	Jones Tender Points
Location	Myofascial, fascial cutaneous, ligamentous, periosteum.	Deep muscle, tendon, ligament, fascia. Often found in the tissue on site opposite site of pain.
Pain Patterns	Referred pain pattern. Patient not usually aware of these sore spots.	Local tenderness, exquisite.
Treatment Position	Direct Technique: Stretch.	Indirect Technique: Shorten tissues.
Onset	Sudden onset during or shortly following acute overload stress or a history of gradual onset secondary to chronic overload of the affected muscle.	Usually acute: Quite often no apparent reason other than changing position quickly.
Types	Active, latent, secondary, satellite, primary, associated, myofascial Trigger Points.	Points generally named for the involved tissue, i.e., (a) Anterior T-12 or those tissues located in the anterior flexor side of the 12th thoracic vertebra; (b) Extended Ankle Tender Point (EXA) located in the gastrocnemius muscle, which extends the ankle; (c) iliacus, serratus anterior or coronal tender points: those points located in a muscle, at an insertion, or on a suture.
Symptoms	With active trigger points, pain projects to a reference zone.	On palpation these points are exquisitely tender but refer no pain.
Multiplicity	Can perpetuate indirectly in other tissues.	Can perpetuate secondary to efferent overflow and gamma gain in a chronically facilitated segment.
ROM	Loss of active/passive range of motion noted. Postural changes evident.	Loss of active/passive range of motion noted. Postural changes evident.
Strength	Decreased with acute or latent trigger points.	Decreased; potential for atrophy.
Synonyms Names*	Spray and Stretch, Trigger Point Therapy, Travell's Trigger Points.	Counterstrain, Strain and Counterstrain, Hold and Fold, Positioning for Comfort, Positional Release, Indirect Technique.

*Not to be confused with Chapman's Reflexes or Motor Points.

CHAPTER 12

A NON-LINEAR APPROACH TO CONNECTIVE TISSUE INTEGRATION
THE SYSTEMS

An Integrated Systems Approach

It has often been stated by many of our mentors, either directly or indirectly, that you cannot recognize what you have not heard of or don't know! (Lowen and Weiselfish 1996; Korr 1975; Guyton 1986; Now, Holmes, and Law 1984). The authors of this text have quite often responded to this wisdom by demonstrating new learning to colleagues in seminars around the world and to patients who are taking part in their own recovery process. When communicating connective tissue concepts, especially in the face of our seminar participants' baseline knowledge regarding this new learning, we have encountered a few problems. There was a failure to recognize the possibility of utilizing the body's full array of connective tissues for healing. Myofascial release constructs were limiting our colleagues' potential. There was a failure to integrate additional structures and systems within the treatment regimen, limiting the possibility of facilitating a greater total body response.

Some practitioners argue that using this approach—treating multiple systems—is far too encompassing to be specific enough to treat local pathology. We emphasize, however, that acknowledgment and treatment of many systems simultaneously can be coupled with an accurate assessment of the local dysfunctional problems and processes. Recovery is actually attained far faster than with conventional single-system approaches. For example, traditional *thoracic outlet syndrome* tests attempt to localize pathology, generally at the *scalene, costoclavicular articulation,* or the *pectoralis minor,* where the *brachial plexus* is often compressed. When the total connective tissue panorama and all other systems are considered, restrictions that can mimic thoracic outlet syndrome may come directly from many different structures. We have found such restrictions within the spinal cord *(spinal fibrosis),* *extradural restrictions* (between the cord and dura), restrictions at the *dural sleeve,* both from within the sleeve (between the nerve root and the inside of the sleeve) and external to the sleeve (between the sleeve and surrounding tissues), *extra-neural restrictions* (between the nerve trunk, root, cord and surrounding tissues) and *intraneural restrictions* (within the fibers of the nerve itself). We have also noted restrictions lateral to the pectoralis minor at the *glenoid labrum,* and as far away as the carpal tunnel and palmer fascia. The latter two sites are usually part of a double or triple crush phenomena and consistently contribute to thoracic outlet problems. Utilizing a multisystems approach during manual assessment makes it is possible to be very specific and at the same time alert to the possible involvement of other, interrelated systems. For example, we can ask: is there inflammation? In other words, is there dysfunction of the circulation/lymphatic systems? Is there muscle spasm? In other words, is there dysfunction of the neurologic and muscle systems? Is there a postural or ergonomic problem? In other words, is there dysfunction of the neuromusculoskeletal system? Is there a fascial problem? In other words, is there dysfunction of the visceral and connective/fascia tissue systems? Is there an emotional problem being manifested in a physical system? In other words, is there dysfunction of the energetic system e.g., the acupuncture meridian system or body-mind system)? Are there symptoms that don't correlate with dermatomes, myotomes, scleratomes, enterotomes—for example, the dura of the craniosacral system? Are there vascular changes, i.e., changes in the cardiac, respiratory, or autonomic nervous systems? Many of these symptoms can be reviewed in isolation, as will be delineated in the rest of this chapter, but in reality they should be assessed in relation to the rest of the body's functions.

In acknowledgement of the many forms of connective tissue in the greater picture of the body, we present a system-by-system review. We will attempt to highlight salient components.

The Skeletal System

Calling bone the building block and supportive framework for the rest of the body is, at times, actually something of an overstatement. Bone itself is classified as a supporting tissue, but must be viewed in the light of the other connective tissues and systems which help support *it* (Lowen 1990). Erect posture, for instance, is not achieved by stacking bones, as if block upon block. There are very few "square" bones upon which such stacking might occur. The position of the bones is directly correlated, in most cases, with the soft tissue/connective tissue attached to them. For example, the authors' view of partial *idiopathic scoliosis* is that it is not an isolated skeletal anomaly but a manifestation of abnormal soft tissue forces sustained physically for extended periods of time. This is possible because bones, as well as soft tissues, can retain the impact of stresses and strains within their matrix/ground substance, and this can lead to altered physiology. This also means that with appropriate positioning and techniques, a skilled therapist can facilitate changes in osseous structures affected with scoliotic curvatures (Kain 1996; Hall 1992; Upledger 1995; Netter 1989).

The Muscle System

We have alluded to the many components of connective tissue and their forms within this system. From the level of the myofibril (multiple *sarcomeres*) and its enclosure by the endomysium, to the fascicle, which is surrounded by perimysium, to the muscle, which is encased in epimysium, connective tissue acts as a barrier, facilitator, shock absorber, coordinator of movement, and integrator of information. These individual layers are connected by additional connective tissue and are surrounded by external layers of sheets of thick fascia (Cantu and Grodin1992; Hukins 1984; Calliet 1988; Lowen 1990). These thicker, or at times thinner, layers extend beyond localized quadrants. Via fascia, the head is truly connected to the foot! Tendons, as stated previously, are the extensions of the two outer layers of the muscle fascia. The attachment of tendons and ligaments to bones occurs in a graded fashion, which exposes the soft tissue to increased potential for breakdown, due to stark changes in the viscoelastic properties of the tendons and ligaments as they transition onto and into bone.

The Ligament System

The ligaments, although classified as dense regular connective tissue, comprise a system of interactive supports that can be assessed locally at a joint, or in relation to all of the ligaments of the body in a kinetic chain.

The Endocrine System

The major components of this system are obviously glandular, yet connective tissues play a key role in the physiology of each of the system's structures, individually as well as in functional units. There are specific fascial envelopes of the pancreas, thyroid, thymus, adrenals, heart, testes, digestive glands, kidneys, hypothalamus, pituitary gland, parathyroid, ovaries, and pineal gland exist that are all accessible to manual forces via direct and indirect fascial approaches. Barral, Lowen, Upledger and (Weiselfish) Giammatteo utilize biomechanical as well as mechanoenergetic interfaces to normalize tensions, restrictions, adhesions, fixations, and pressures with various manual approaches (Barral 1988; Barral 1991; Hoffa 1900; Berquist and Shaw 1978). Because structure

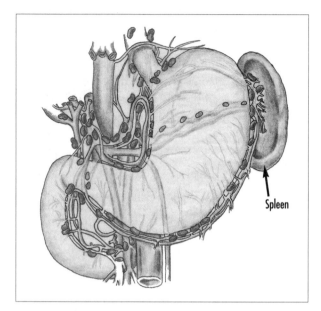

Figure 18a. Spleen.

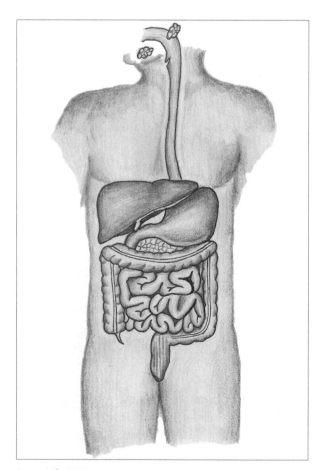

Figure 18b. Digestive system.

does affect function and fascial connections exist in all structures and layers of the body, a working familiarity with the gross and fine anatomy of the endocrine system is warranted. The interventions that can affect these tissues, e.g., visceral mobilization, cranial therapy, and other methods should be studied.

The Lymphatic System

This system comprises some of the most important connective tissue in the entire body. Without a functioning lymphatic system we would be dead within twenty-four hours. The lymph itself is, of course, classified as a fluid connective tissue (Lowen 1990). A close look at a lymph node and at lymph chains in the interstitium will reveal the intimacy between the lymphatic system and connective tissue proper and highlight their respective roles. (See Figure 18a.) The lymphatic system, by the way, also includes the spleen and thymus, both of which can be affected directly by visceral approaches. The nodes are comprised of connective tissue sheaths and reticular fibers. Certain lymph vessels course deeply through the body along with arteries and veins. Lymph flow is closely associated with the health of the circulatory and muscle system, i.e., *structure dictates function*. The lymph vessels (approximately 40 percent of them are found superficially in the skin [Wittlinger and Wittlinger 1982] and subcutaneous tissues) play an important role in drainage and waste removal, as well as in maintaining homeostasis at the level of the superficial fascia.

The Digestive System

This system extends from the mouth to the anus (similar to the endocrine system) and is dominated by glands, the *biliary system*, and pancreas. Hollow organs facilitate the transport, digestion, absorption, and elimination of foodstuffs. Within the linings of these many structures there is loose connective tissue.

We can intervene with therapy via manipulation of the fascial envelopes surrounding these organs according to the practice of Barral and Chauffour, and we can more directly affect the parenchyma more directly applying the practice of Lowen, (Weiselfish) Giammatteo. (See Figure 18b.)

Visceral Manipulation as developed by Jean Pierre Barral (Barral 1993; Weiselfish 1981) focuses on the restoration of mobility and motility (Barral 1991) of the organs, specifically the fascial envelopes. Barral found that all organs have an inherent circadian motion, which he characterizes as motility. The balance between mobility and motility is greatly affected by fascial restrictions, either local or distal to the organ. Barral's knowledge of biomechanics and his research using various high technology diagnostic tools have facilitated the validation of his approach. Clinically, Dr. Barral has over 55,000 case studies at his disposal for research purposes. Barral discerned lines of tension associated with patterns of fascial restrictions.

Paralleling Barral's work, Paul Chauffour elaborated on the mobilization of viscera with Mechanical Link. (Weiselfish) Giammatteo contributed an approach to restore the normal dimensions of the spaces between organs and normalize internal organ pressures, and Lowen focused on intervisceral parenchymal cell motility.

The Respiratory System

This system encompasses all passageways from the nasal cavities to the lungs. Connective tissue components here include the cartilages in the trachea; all craniofacial fascial interrelationships; the fascial linings (know as *pleura* in the lungs) covering the lung tissue proper; the inside of the thoracic cavity; and the *mediastinum,* which is the fascia that covers the trachea, the esophagus, and which heats and lines the medial aspect of the lungs. (See Figures 19a to 19c.) Additionally, the fascial nature of the diaphragm is integral to the

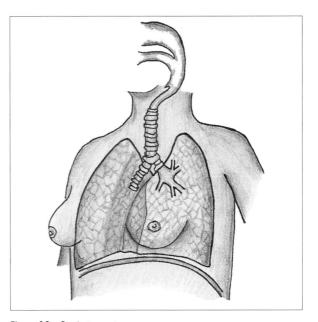

Figure 19a. Respiratory system.

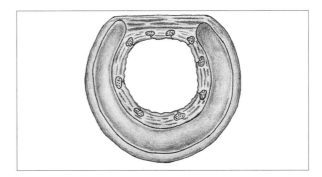

Fugure 19b. Transverse cross-section of trachea.

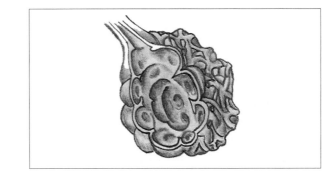

Figure 19c. Aveolar structure.

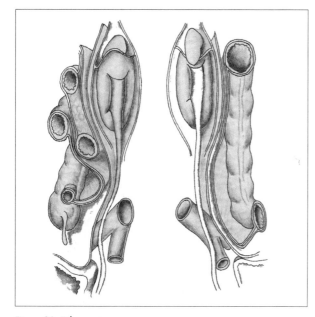

Figure 20. Kidney system.

respiratory, circulatory, and digestive systems. The fascial envelopes of the diaphragms together with their physiologic functions create a sub-atmospheric pressure within the thorax (Barral 1991). The baseline pressure is approximately -5 cm H$_2$O. This pressure can rise according to pressures generated by coughing, sneezing, *valsalvas,* trauma, etc. This subatmospheric pressure has a direct effect of the contents of the thorax, both biomechanically and physiologically, and has an indirect effect on the contents of the abdomen. Because of the pull of the sub-atmospheric pressure upwards, the relative weight of the abdominal organs is less than without this pressure. Secondary to this phenomenon, ligaments and fascia within both the thoracic and abdominal cavities have altered components and roles. First, visceral ligaments are much less tensile than ligaments of the musculoskeletal system. They act more like tethers than stabilizers. They also help coordinate movement similar to the peripheral ligaments. Fascial mobility between the pleural layers of the lungs, i.e., the *visceral* and *parietal pleurae,* is essential for lung mobility while head, neck, and chest postural alignment is also greatly affected by this mobility. Without adequate mobil-

ity between the two layers, subsequent irritation of surrounding soft tissues, including the lungs, is likely even when the restriction is small. Movement excursions via the diaphragm are significant. The diaphragm excursion of 24,000 breaths per day at 3 cm in inhalation and exhalation yields approximately 600 meters of motion. Imagine what fascial restriction, capable of causing an altered axis of motion, would do to any of the surrounding tissues.

The Reproductive/Kidney System

These systems are reviewed together because their relationships to connective tissue are similar. The kidneys, uterus, bladder, prostate, and ovaries are encased in layers of fascia that can be used as handles to facilitate soft tissue balance in those areas (Barral 1991). (See Figure 20.) Because of the interconnectedness of the fascial tissues, the *pelvic bowl* fascias are directly connected to the neck and cranium.

The Circulatory System

Blood as a fluid connective tissue has been discussed previously. In addition, blood vessels have a significant connective tissue component. Collagen alone accounts for 20 percent of the dry weight of the large elastic arteries and 50 percent of smaller vessels (Frankel and Nordin 1980). Type I and III collagen make up most of this collagen. Other types of collagen have also been found, including Type IV, V, VI and VIII, plus one similar to Type X, and an additional kind of collagen with elastic fibers. Each type of collagen plays a specific role in the function of the vessel wall (Frankel and Nordin 1980). On a larger scale, there are three distinct layers of the blood vessels (artery or vein): the tunica externa, tunica media, and tunica interna. The interna layer is dominated by elastic fibers; the externa layer anchors itself to surrounding tissues (Lowen 1990).

The heart contains an outer connective

tissue layer surrounded by the fascial layer of the pericardium. The pericardium is actually a layer of dense fibrous connective tissue on top of a loose connective tissue layer. The heart proper has three layers of muscle tissue similar to peripheral muscle tissue, vascular tissue, and nerve tissue: (1) *epicardium,* (2) *myocardium,* and (3) *endocardium,* with layers of loose connective tissue interposed.

The Nervous System

This complex system will be considered regarding the peripheral and the central nervous systems respectively.

There are three layers of connective tissue recognized in the peripheral nerve complex. The inner layer, the *endoneurium,* surrounds a collagenous basement membrane. It is elastic by nature, with a matrix of capillaries, collagen, fibroblasts, mast cells, and *Schwann cells.* This tissue helps maintain pressures within this level of the nerve. The second layer is the *perineurium,* which is the layer apparently most responsible for offsetting tensile forces (Butler 1991) from the nerve. The outermost layer of connective tissue is the *epineurium,* which protects and cushions the inner structure of the nerve. This layer actually has an internal and external component. Unlike the blood vessels that anchor their outer layer to surrounding tissues, the epineurium makes the nerve quite distinct from surrounding tissues. Butler (Butler 1991) sites another loose areolar tissue called *mesoneurium* around the peripheral nerve trunks. This tissue must remain mobile at all time. It has been noted that blood vessels enter the nerve via various channels.

The connective tissues of the central nervous system are integral to its mechanical support as well as to its protection. They are also essential in the maintenance of nutrient transportation and blood and fluid circulation (Weiss 1984). The outermost layer of the brain and spinal cord, the dura mater, provides an adequate transition from the soft, semi-solid brain to the inner aspects of the cranium. The existence of connective tissues in the form of the dura, pia, and arachnoid membranes, plus loose connective tissue, indicate the importance of all the brain structure's individual functions.

All of the body's fascial tissues, inclusive of the reciprocal tension membranes, anchor at the *foramen magnum.*

After this review, connective tissue's ubiquitous nature should be evident. Every system is intimately connected with and exists among these tissues. It is time for all manual practitioners to rethink their positions on what we think we know, what we could know, and what we should know.

CHAPTER 13

MYOFASCIAL DYSFUNCTION
THE PATHOPHYSIOLOGY OF INTERDEPENDENT TISSUES AND ORGANS

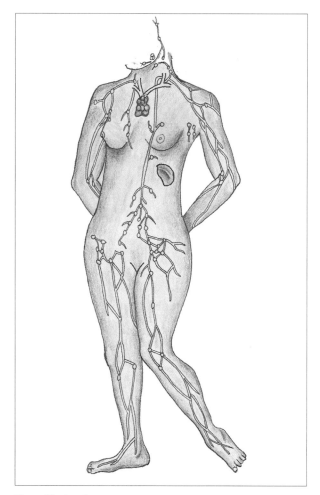

Figure 21a. Lymphatic system.

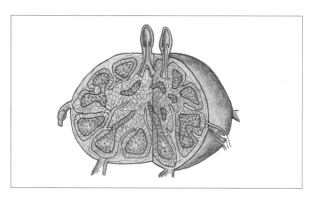

Figure 21b. Lymph node.

The Lymphatic System

The connective tissue system is intricately related with the lymphatic system. (See Figures 21a and 21b.) Typically, when the lymphatic system is discussed, it is done in association with medical problems; for example, cancer or other immune disorders. Yet *lymphatic drainage,* which is the essential function of the lymph system, is a basic physiologic function in its own right. The lymphatic system is also significant as one of the three circulatory systems (together with arterial and venous circulation.)

Many texts cover the basic anatomy and physiology of lymphatic drainage. In this text we present a practical overview.

There are many components of the lymphatic drainage system, in particular: *lymph capillaries, lymph vessels,* and *lymph nodes.* The lymph capillaries absorb all the excess water, protein, fatty acids, and toxins from the ground substance of the connective tissue (i.e., the waste products of the cells). This absorbed content, the *lymph load,* is processed through the lymph nodes, which are purification centers. The lymph nodes disperse the toxic content to the liver for further detoxification. Toxins are then filtered through the kidneys and lower bowels for excretion. Traversing through the lymph nodes are the chains of lymph vessels, which are fine, silk-like vessels, found in the skin (40 percent) and in deeper tissue (60 percent).

Muscles innervated by the autonomic nervous system are present in each lymph vessel. When these muscles contract, the lymph load is pushed into the neighboring lymph vessels. The lymph load is processed through the body towards the heart. By the time the lymph load reaches the heart, if the lymph nodes are healthy, the residual content, which is projected into the heart, will have been purified. There should not be any toxic affect on the heart. Essentially, elimination of all the toxins in the connective tissue matrix, the ground substance, is dependent on the lymphatic system.

The lymph load of the legs drains into the *cistern chyle* in the abdomen. The abdominal lymph load will be processed through the cistern chyle as well. From the cistern chyle, the excess lymph load will continue into the *thoracic duct*. At the superior aspect of the thoracic duct, drainage from the left arm, the left of the face, head, and neck and a small portion of the lung comes together. This lymph load, approximately 75 percent of the total body lymphatic drainage, will be processed through the left *terminus* in the thoracic inlet, into the *superior vena cava*, and from there into the *right atrium* of the heart. The rest of the body's lymph load to be drained from most of the lungs, the right arm, the right of the face, head, and neck, will drain through the right terminus in the right thoracic inlet, in to the superior vena cava and then the heart.

INTEGRATIVE MANUAL THERAPY
Left Thoracic Inlet Syndrome is more severe than on the right side, because 75 percent of the total body lymphatic drainage is processed through the left terminus at the left thoracic inlet. This means that 75 percent of total body congestion can result secondary to Left Thoracic Inlet Syndrome.
Clinically, the following signs are evident to observers: legs, abdomen, left leg, left arm, the left of the head, left of the neck, and face will be edematous with left thoracic inlet dysfunction; chest, right arm, right of the head, neck, and face will be edematous with right thoracic inlet dysfunction.

The association between connective tissue proper and lymphatic tissue is a form of interdependence. All metabolic processes will be dependent for rate of transport, quality of transport, and quantity of transport, on the lymphatic drainage of waste, toxins, excess protein, amino acids, and water via the ground substance. When lymphatic drainage is not functional, there is a build up of wastes and proteins in the matrix, which causes a destabilization of the ground substance. Fibrosis will begin within hours of the onset of poor lymphatic drainage. This fibrosis will continue as a hyperreactive process until stabilization returns. This cannot happen until good lymphatic drainage is restored.

INTEGRATIVE MANUAL THERAPY
A process of degeneration of the ground substance occurs secondary to poor lymphatic drainage, causing fibrosis, fibromyalgia, myositis, myofibrositis, fibromyositis, and other conditions.

The Liver and Related Tissues: Detoxification

The liver is the most significant detoxification center of the body. (See Figure 22.) Proteins are deformed and transformed for excretion. Toxins are excreted either transformed or in original form. All of the toxins are already detoxified to some degree by the time the liver can access them. Toxins pass via lymph nodes through the lymph vessels. The lymph nodes process the toxins. Then they are further processed in the liver. From the liver, toxins are dispersed through the process of *kidney detoxification*. This is particularly true for many water-soluble substances. Whatever is not processed via the liver will be returned to the ground substance. When the liver is edematous, inflamed, or degenerating, the toxic content cannot be processed. Unprocessed toxins, when returned to the ground substance, influence the fibrolytic process, which becomes hyperactive with inflammation. All of the longer proteins and long-chain fatty acids contribute to this inflammation, returning to the matrix when they should be eliminated. This inflammation will be perpetuated and

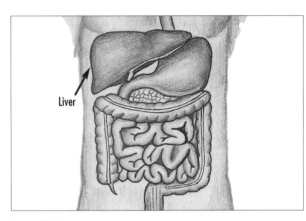

Figure 22. Liver.

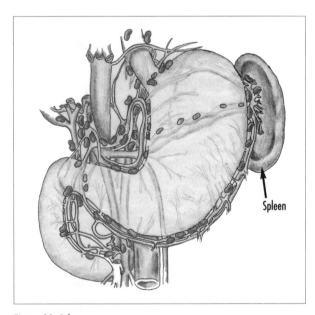

Figure 23. Spleen.

can spread throughout the total body matrix, affecting organs, tissues, and other structures, which can become inflamed in turn (e.g., manifesting as *periarthritis, pericarditis, meningitis, osteoarthritis,* and other conditions). Poor liver function will cause some degree of this metastatic-like process to occur, whenever toxins, proteins, and fatty-acids are not processed for excretion.

The Spleen and Its Affect On Other Connective Tissue Function

The spleen is an immune system organ, yet it is also a component structure of the connective tissue system. (See Figure 23.) A healthy spleen is necessary for fibrolysis and for demolition of fibrotic material. Antibodies, especially *T-cells,* are macrophages for anticonnective tissue cells. When an *autoimmune deficiency* is present, there can be a low collagen to elastin ratio. Systemic hypermobility will be evident (e.g., capsular and ligamentous laxity and hyperflexibility of the soft tissue, muscles, and connective tissue). When an immunodeficiency is present, a response more sever than systemic hypermobility can also occur within the connective tissue system. Proliferation of connective tissue fibers and cells (hyplasia) will occur, which is similar to a malalignment-like process. In cases of autoimmune hyperactivity, as in rheumatoid arthritis, there is an exacerbation of macrophagic activity, destroying connective tissue cells and fibers.

All of the spleen's functions are interdependent with immune system functions. There is an interdependence of the connective tissue system with the whole of the immune system.

The Heart and Related Tissues: Lymph and Connective Tissue Interface

The heart is a major source of energy for the connective tissue system. Lymph, produced in the heart, is plasma-like in content, and is the carrier of the entire lymph load through the chains of lymph vessels, which finally return the lymph to the heart for reprocessing. When the heart is functioning poorly, it will forego some of its essential tasks, including the production of lymph. With this lowering of lymph-count, there will be inefficient lymphatic drainage, causing a build-up of toxins, proteins, water, and fatty acids in the ground substance, resulting in fibrosis of the ground substance, organs, muscles, and nerves. (See Figure 24.)

For lymph production, oxygen is essential; therefore, all disorders affecting oxygenation in the heart will contribute to a lowering of the lymph count.

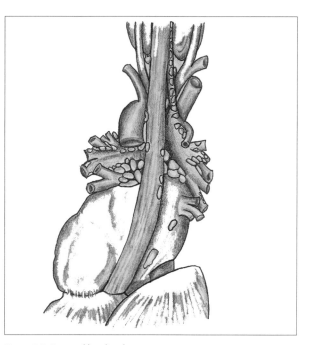

Figure 24. Heart and lymph nodes.

PART THREE

THE TECHNIQUES OF MYOFASCIAL RELEASE:
A 3-PLANAR FASCIAL FULCRUM APPROACH

CHAPTER 14

THE CLINICAL PRACTICE OF MYOFASCIAL RELEASE
GENERAL CONSIDERATIONS

When Myofascial Release is the Treatment of Choice

There are many problems for which the manual treatment of body may be appropriate. These problems can be structural, functional, or both structural and functional. When the problem is structural, there may be a combination of any of the following: *joint hypomobility, connective tissue dysfunction, muscle fiber hypertonicity or atrophy, fascial dysfunction, neural tissue tensions, organ dysfunction, circulatory dysfunction, periosteal tension, ligamentous problems, tendon dysfunction, capsule tissue length/tension pressures,* and other conditions. When the problems are functional, there may be a combination of any of the following: weakness, imbalance, disequilibria, loss of coordination, *proprioception compromise, exteroception loss, apraxia,* cognition compromise, visual perceptual problems, and other symptoms.

We have arrived at the conclusion that *structural rehabilitation* and *functional rehabilitation* can be treated as separate categories for the purpose of organizing therapeutic intervention. "Structural rehabilitation" specifically denotes therapy for the correction of *pathoanatomy, pathophysiology, pathomechanics,* and *pathoenergy.* "Functional rehabilitation" refers to functional outcome. It is concerned with whether the client is able to function optimally in all activities of daily living.

The categories of structural and functional rehabilitation can be further delineated. Structure includes many systems so that manual therapy can be made specific to address healing on a cellular level. The requirements for the healing of anatomic components differ for each system. Joint biomechanics, muscles, connective tissue, nervous tissue, organ, cell, blood vessel, and other systems are different in their macroscopic and microscopic aspects. Function is delineated according to requirements for activities of daily living: strength, balance, coordination, exteroception, proprioception, and other functions. Healing techniques for different body systems have been developed and collected over the past twenty years. Approaches to facilitate function according to particular functional impairments have been compiled and evolved during that time. The combined processes of structural rehabilitation and functional rehabilitation comprise Integrative Manual Therapy. Myofascial Release is the treatment of choice when *structural* dysfunction exists within the connective tissue system.

The Integrated Systems Approach

It is often effective and efficient to assess the specific anatomic tissue and/or structure that is unhealthy, and to use a system-specific approach to therapy. If the problem is within the muscle fiber, the approach of choice might be a technique that can eliminate hypertonicity (for example, Strain and Counterstrain Technique, as developed by Jones). When the problem is within the joint space, often joint mobilizations (Mennell, Paris, Kaltenborn, Maitland) or Muscle Energy and Beyond Technique (Mitchell, then ((Weiselfish)) Giammatteo) is a more appropriate therapeutic intervention. When the problem is within the tissues of the brain and/or spinal cord, cranial therapies are effective and efficient methods of intervention. If the problem is inherent within the connective tissue system, Myofascial Release will be the most appropriate choice.

Because the connective tissue ground substance envelops and infiltrates all body tissues and structures, invariably Myofascial Release will attain positive results, no matter which specific system is affected. When the tissues affected are predominantly soft tissues, the Soft Tissue Myofascial Release technique presented in this text will be effective. When the joint biomechanics are dysfunctional, with hyaline cartilage, ligamentous, capsular, and/or tendon compromise, the Articular Myofascial Release technique (present in this text) will almost always attain improved articular balance and increased joint mobility.

Indications, Contraindications, Precautions

Primary *neuromusculoskeletalfascial* dysfunction responds to manual therapies such as Myofascial Release. Whatever problem is being addressed: joint dysfunction, muscle fiber dysfunction, fascial dysfunction, neuronal dysfunction, periosteal and bone dysfunction, circulatory dysfunction, or other conditions, Myofascial Release can be considered as the intervention of choice.

What are the hypothetical primary precautions regarding Myofascial Release, A 3-Planar Fascial Fulcrum Approach? It would seem that, if there is a systemic disorder, Myofascial Release might aggravate the symptoms. According to clinical outcome studies undertaken by these authors, signs will be aggravated in these cases only rarely. For instance, if there is cancer, it might be feared that metastasis would be promoted. There is, however, no clinical indication to date that supports this concern. Again, if there is nonunion of a fracture, Myofascial Release might be feared to cause further displacement of the bony ends of the fracture sites. Typically, however, union is promoted with Myofascial Release. Again, no clinical evidence exists to support this concern. Finally, if there is congestive heart failure, one might expect that an increase in venous and lymphatic return to the heart might compromise the patient's well-being. This too has been found not to be the case in clinical research.

In almost fifteen years of clinical practice, no real contraindications to the 3-Planar Fascial Fulcrum Approach have been discovered. We have treated many varied patient populations with it, including pediatric, geriatric, neurologic, cardiac, respiratory, chronic pain, orthopedic, sports medicine, systemic illness, cancer, and other populations. We have treated acute and chronic patients. We have performed pre- and post-surgical interventions with this technique. Results have been consistent whether looked at according to diagnosis, age, chronicity, severity, or nature of illness and disorder.

When practical, thoughtful, considerate therapy is practiced, negative side effects are not commonly induced. Unwanted treatment reaction is more likely to be the result of change in posture, body mechanics, joint and soft tissue mobility, and movement than directly induced by the approach itself.

Manual Therapy and Fascial/Myofascial Dysfunction

Neuromusculoskeletal dysfunction causes postural dysfunction. Postural dysfunction produces fascial tensions. The traction and compression produced by postural dysfunction upon the sensory nerve elements and free nerve endings within the connective tissue system often cause pain.

As the manual therapist develops the specialized sense of touch necessary for diagnosis of tissue disorders, differential diagnosis is facilitated. An educated tactile sense can determine if tissue is tense, relaxed, or altered due to an imbalance of tissue chemistry. The development of palpation skills is essential for the accurate diagnosis of fascial dysfunction.

Fascial dysfunction can contribute to changes in local, regional, and total body health. Ligamentous tension alterations are important in joint lesion pathology. The stretching of ligaments can result in the *hypermobility of joints. Ligament adhesions* compromise intra-articular and extra-articular tissues and structures. *Subluxations* and *dislocations of bone,* whether mild with imbalance of the articular surfaces, or severe, result in tendon tension. This tendon tension is transmitted to muscle fibers, which produce compensatory hypertonicity and sustained muscle contractions.

Immobilization may result in fascial dysfunction. Research has provided evidence that long periods of immobilization produce muscle atrophy, joint stiffness, *ulceration of joint cartilage,* osteoarthritis, *skin necrosis,* infection, *tendocutaneous adhesion, thrombophlebitis,* and varying degrees of contracture. Research has provided evidence that synovial fluid, post immobilization, has excessive connective tissue deposition in the joint and joint recesses (e.g., *heterotopic ossification*). Chronic and excessive deposition of fibrous connective tissue forms mature scars and creates intra-articular adhesions. Postimmobilization matrix changes have been reported in ligament, capsule, tendon, and fascia. Studies show that controlled passive mobilization promotes gliding and accelerates the healing rate of tendons. With immobilization, reports of water loss, increased synthesis of new collagen, and an increase in the cross-links between collagen fibers have been presented. This excessive and abnormal cross-link formation between fibers contributes to joint restriction, yet research has also provided evidence that *functional loading* can cause *regeneration* of tendons.

In order to explain the results of the 3-Planar Fascial Fulcrum Approach to Myofascial Release, a hypothetical model based on energy is presented. The authors extrapolate from the understanding of *quanta.* They present the medium for this fascial release technique as energy and apply the theories of particle and wave motion presented in the scientific field of quantum physics.

Myofascial Release

What is Myofascial Release? It is a treatment modality that focuses on dysfunction within the connective tissue system. The authors believe Myofascial Release has a direct effect on collagen, elastin, the ground substance, and other substances and systems. Fascial dysfunction (connective tissue dysfunction) can be due to physical trauma, inflammation, infection, postural dysfunction, articular restriction, and any external or internal body torsion that contributes to fascial strain.

If the fascia has shortened and tightened and twisted, it can contribute to and perpetuate neuromusculoskeletal dysfunction. Myofascial Release techniques are assumed to affect the continuous, contiguous, connective tissue system that envelops every cell and fiber in the body. The goal is to relieve fascial restrictions and to normalize the health and tension of this body system. Myofascial Release apparently affects the *elastacollagenous complex* (integrated collagen and elastin fibers), as well as the consistency of the ground substance. Increased soft-tissue flexibility relieves tissue tension within the elastocollagenous complex. While the density and viscosity of the matrix (ground substance) decreases, the metabolic rate increases, resulting in improved metabolism and health.

The direction of fascial release can be *direct* or *indirect.* (See next section.) This 3-Planar Fascial Fulcrum approach is always indirect. Treatment is more comfortable than with direct methods. Body resistance is less when little or no force is applied to engage barriers. The initial mechanical forces of Myofascial Release are transcribed into an energy force at the *mechanoenergetic interface.* The energy flow affects the viscoelastic properties of the fascia.

The concept of the *fulcrum* is significant for these reasons: (1) A fulcrum is a *fixed point* around which the tissues can unravel and unwind. This process of *pressure unwinding* attains soft tissue flexibility. (2) A fulcrum is a mechanoenergetic interface where energy is (hypothetically) created, transduced, or transformed. Although Newton hypothesized that energy cannot be created or destroyed, there is some research evidence that suggests that energy *can* be created under certain controlled circumstances. But whether or not energy is actually created at the fulcrum, there is no question but that the fulcrum is a mechanoenergetic interface where energy is transduced and transmitted.

The development of palpation skills facilitates the diagnosis of fascial dysfunction. The observation of postural asymmetry, the palpation of fascial glide and mobility, and Myofascial Mapping are relatively easy assessment tools for the manual practitioner to develop.

Direct and Indirect Techniques

Manual therapy in general comprises direct and indirect techniques. Direct techniques *load* or *bind* tissue and structures. The tissue is moved *towards* a barrier on one or more planes. The direction of displacement of the tissue is in the least mobile, most restricted, most limited direction. The technique is performed at or just before the barrier. The result is a change of the position of the barrier, which will move closer to what would be the end of a more normal range of motion. For example, if there is an *elbow flexion contracture* with contracted and shortened biceps and a limitation of elbow extension, a direct technique would move the elbow into extension. At the barrier, or just before the barrier at the *interbarrier zone,* a technique is performed. The result is an increased range of extension motion.

Indirect techniques *unload* or *ease* the tissue and structures. The tissue is moved *away* from the barrier on one or more planes. The direction of movement of the tissue is in the most mobile, least restricted, least limited direction. The distortion is thereby exacerbated. The problem is exaggerated. For example, if the problem is limited extension, there is relatively too much flexion. The problem could be described as *excessive flexion.* The treatment would be towards flexion. The result is a "release" phenomenon: the soft tissues "let go" of tension in a *tissue tension release.* This permits an increased range of motion past the original barrier. For example, if there is an elbow flexion contracture with contracted and

shortened biceps and a limitation of elbow extension, the elbow would be moved into flexion. A "release" phenomenon occurs by the end of the technique, resulting in decreased hypertonicity, increased elongation of the biceps, and increased range of extension motion.

Myofascial Release techniques are more effective, more efficient, less aggressive to the client, and involve less energy expenditure on the part of the therapist when they are performed as indirect techniques.

Tissue-Tension Release

The practitioner monitors tissue tension throughout the duration of the manual therapy technique. When tissue tension changes, softens, and relaxes, this is a "tissue-tension release." These releases occur during the treatment with Myofascial Release.

This decrease in tissue tension during manual therapy has been attributed to several factors. One factor is the decrease in *efferent neuron activity (gamma and alpha impulses)* resulting in a decreased resistance of the *muscle spindle,* and the relaxation and elongation of the sarcomere. Another factor is the change of elastic resistance to viscous compliance of the soft tissue due to morphologic changes. There is an apparent relaxation of the elastic fibers during a release. Tissue-tension release occurs together with a perception of increased fluid and increased energy throughout the tissues. During the treatment technique, heat emanates from involved body tissues. There is a sensation of movement, a filling of space, and often a *therapeutic pulse.*

This therapeutic pulse occurs frequently during manual therapy in general and Myofascial Release techniques in particular. The amplitude of force of this therapeutic pulse increases during the treatment technique and subsides as the tissue tension releases and as the technique is completed.

CHAPTER 15

THE SOFT TISSUE MYOFASCIAL RELEASE TECHNIQUE

There are two primary forms of Myofascial Release: the technique for soft tissue and the technique for joints. The protocols for these techniques differ in detail. This chapter presents the method for and an example of the soft tissue procedure. Chapter 16 presents the method for and an example of "articular" or "joint" Myofascial Release.

The following are general instructions for the application of Soft Tissue Myofascial Release Technique. The instructions must be adjusted for specific body areas.

INDICATION

Soft Tissue Myofascial Release Technique can be performed when there are the following positive findings. These findings indicate dysfunction:

- Positive Myofascial Mapping
- Decreased fascial glide or compromised fascial mobility
- Joint hypomobility
- Soft tissue tension
- Positive deviations
- Dynamic limitations if ranges of motion.

GENERAL GUIDELINE: A 3-PLANAR CONCEPT
3-Planar Fascial Fulcrum techniques access the body on three planes: sagittal, coronal, and transverse.

APPLICATION

Soft Tissue Myofascial Release Techniques and Articular Fascial Release Techniques can be applied:

- anywhere in the body;
- from proximal to distal;
- from static postural dysfunction to dynamic postural dysfunction;
- from most severe postural dysfunction to least severe postural dysfunction;
- from Soft Tissue Myofascial Release to Articular Fascial Release;
- from superficial fascial layers to deep fascial layers.

TREATMENT

1. "Sandwich" the body part to be treated. Place a hand on either side of the body part.

   Options:

   a. One hand is on the right side, while the second hand is on the left side. (See Figure 25.)

   b. One hand is on the lateral surface while the second hand is on the medial surface. (See Figure 26.)

   c. One hand is on the anterior surface while the second hand is on the posterior surface. (See Figure 27.)

2. Compress the body part with a force of no more than 5 grams. Maintain this compressive force.

3. Move (displace) the tissues: the hands move in opposite directions to each other on three planes.

Distortion of the tissue on the sagittal plane:
Let the hand that is on the anterior surface of the body, move the tissue in a superior direction while the other hand, which is on the posterior surface of the body, moves the tissue in an inferior direction.

Return to neutral and reverse directions: Let the hand that is on the anterior surface of the body move the tissue in an inferior direction, while the other hand, which is on the posterior surface of the body, moves the tissue in a superior direction.

Assess the most mobile distortion (tissue displacement) pattern of the tissues on the sagittal plane. Move the tissues *indirectly* in the direction of ease (greatest tissue mobility, greatest tissue flexibility, least restriction, least inhibition) on this plane.

Distortion of the tissue on the transverse plane:
Let the hand that is on the anterior surface move the tissue in a medial direction while the other hand, which is on the posterior surface of the body, moves the tissue in a lateral direction.

Return to neutral and reverse directions: Let the hand that is on the anterior surface of the body, moves the tissue in a lateral direction, while the other hand, which is on the posterior surface of the body, moves the tissue in a medial direction.

Assess the most mobile distortion (tissue displacement) pattern of the tissues on the transverse plane. Move the tissues *indirectly* in the direction of ease (greatest tissue mobility, greatest tissue flexibility, least restriction, least inhibition) on this plane.

Distortion of the tissue on the coronal plane:
Let the hand that is on the anterior surface of the body move the tissue in a clockwise direction, while the other hand, which is on the posterior surface of the body, moves the tissue in a counter-clockwise direction.

Return to neutral and reverse directions: Let the hand that is on the anterior surface of the body move the tissue in a counter-clockwise direction while the other hand, which is on the posterior surface of the body, moves the tissue in a clockwise direction.

Assess the most mobile distortion (tissue displacement) pattern of the tissues on the coronal plane. Move the tissues *indirectly* in the direction of ease (greatest tissue mobility, greatest tissue flexibility, least restriction, least inhibition) on this plane.

4. Determine the patterns of distortion (tissue displacement) that are the most mobile on each of the three planes. These patterns of tissue distortion were assessed in Step 3. The distortion patterns are those of greatest tissue mobility, greatest tissue flexibility, least restriction, and least inhibition, on all three planes.

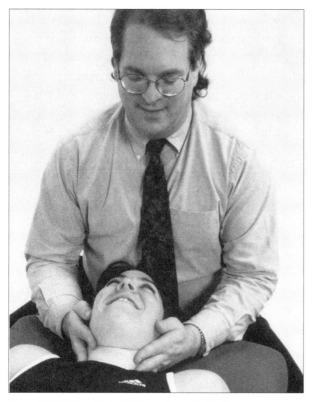

Figure 25. Soft Tissue Myofascial Release: Lateral Neck Hold.

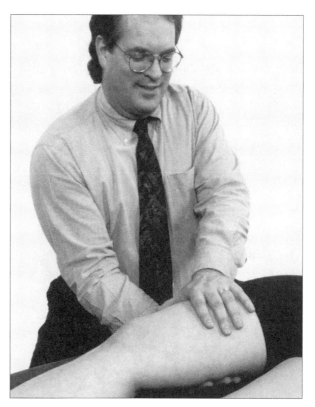

Figure 27. Soft Tissue Myofascial Release over thigh.

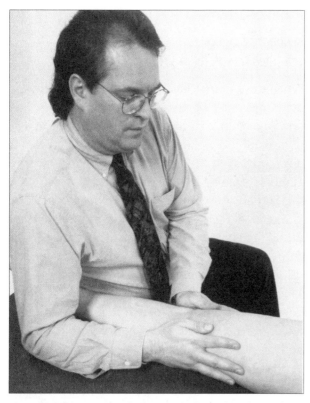

Figure 26. Soft Tissue Myofascial Release: Knee Release. (This technique will access the medial and lateral ligaments as well as the menisci.)

Inhibitory Balance Testing as developed by
Paul Chauffour, D.O. can be utilized between
Steps 4 and 5. Once the therapist is comfortable with
the technique, consider this step to increase
effectiveness and efficiency.

5. Stack the patterns of distortion on all three planes, one plane at a time, according to Inhibitory Balance Process. In the example opposite, the following was determined:

The coronal plane is the most dominant plane. The transverse plane is the second most dominant plane. The sagittal plane is the least dominant plane.

First move the tissue in the mobile pattern of distortion (tissue displacement) on a coronal plane (Step 3). Then move the tissues in the mobile pattern of distortion (tissue displacement) on a transverse plane (Step 3). Then move the tissues in the mobile pattern of distortion (tissue displacement) on a sagittal plane (Step 3).

Note on hand contact: The hands should not move on the skin. Rather, there is a distortion of the internal tissues. Imagine a marshmallow between the two hands. Distort the marshmallow!

6. *The Fulcrum:* There are now four directions of forces from each hand onto the body.

   - Slight compression
   - Coronal plane: clockwise or counter-clockwise
   - Transverse plane: medial or lateral
   - Sagittal plane: superior or inferior

The intersection of these eight forces is a "fixed point." This fixed point is the *fulcrum* around which the fascial tissue will *unwind*. This fulcrum is the mechanoenergetic interface for the 3-Planar Myofascial Fulcrum Technique.

7. *Tissue Tension Release:* Maintain the fulcrum. The hands do not move. They do not follow the tissue movements, although the temptation to move the hands and

follow the tissue motion will be great. The goal is not a physiologic unwinding of a body part. The objective is the internal "unraveling" of the fascial tissue. By maintaining the fulcrum, energy will be created/transduced. The force of the energy causing the fascial release will produce more changes in the internal environment of the connective tissue. The fascial unwinding will be slow and gentle. Do not allow quick or repetitive or forceful physiologic movements.

If the patient begins to move any body part quickly, without repetition, or with force, say to the patient: "Please don't move in that manner." If the body part changes position in space slowly and gently in order to facilitate the internal tissue unwinding, this movement is acceptable. At the end of the release, the hands will be in different positions because of the unwinding of the internal body tissues. The body parts that experienced the internal tissue unwinding will be in a more normal anatomical, neutral position.

Inhibitory Balance Testing and Inhibitory Balance Process

When the 3-Planar Fascial Fulcrum Approach was developed in 1981, stacking of the planes was done according to the mobile pattern of distortion on all three planes. At that time, planes were not compared for dominance. In 1994, the authors began to study with Paul Chauffour, D.O, the French osteopathic physician and developer of a manual therapy approach called "Mechanical Link." This procedure investigates multiple systems: joints of the upper and lower extremities, spine, rib cage, cranium, and other systems. The Mechanical Link investigation includes a "nullification" process, in order to determine what is the dominant system and primary problem in the body. Once the problem is discovered, treatment applied is called "Recoil." It is a direct approach to mobilization. Dr. Chauffour has allowed us to

Inhibitory Balance Testing

The purpose of Inhibitory Balance Testing (IBT) is to determine the best order for treatment. Perform IBT to compare which plane—sagittal, coronal, or transverse—is more *dominant* or *primary*.

An example:

1. Compare sagittal plane with transverse plane:
   a. Move the tissues in the chosen direction of ease on a sagittal plane. In other words, move the tissues superior or inferior (because MFR is *indirect,* travel in the direction of least resistance). Let's assume that the chosen direction on a sagittal plane is superior.
   b. While maintaining the tissues in superior glide, now "stack on" movement of the tissues in the chosen direction of ease on a transverse plane. In other words, while the tissues are in a superior direction, stack on medial or lateral glide. Let's assume medial was the direction of transverse plane movement that was added to the fulcrum.
   c. Once medial glide (transverse plane) has been added to the fascial fulcrum, test if there is greater movement potential than before on a sagittal plane. In other words, now that the tissues have been moved in superior glide to the limitation and then medial glide to the limitation, test if there is greater movement in superior glide.

Question:
Did the transverse plane movement (medial glide) *affect* the sagittal plane movement (superior glide)? Did movement in superior glide increase? Did the initial limitation on a sagittal plane increase once the distortion on a transverse plane was added?

Answer:
YES. Superior glide increased. Tissue displacement on a sagittal plane increased when the transverse plane was added. The tissue on a sagittal plane was less resistant to distortion. —*or*—
NO. Superior glide did not increase. Tissue displacement on a sagittal plane did not increase when the transverse plane was added. The limitation on a sagittal plane remained the same.

Conclusion:
If the answer is YES (transverse plane *did affect* movement on a sagittal plane), then transverse plane is dominant to sagittal plane.
If the answer is NO (transverse plane *did not affect* movement on a sagittal plane), then transverse plane is not dominant to sagittal plane. In fact, sagittal plane is dominant to transverse plane.

Application for Treatment:
If transverse plane is dominant to sagittal plane, then transverse plane should be stacked prior to sagittal plane.
If sagittal plane is dominant to transverse plane, then sagittal plane should be stacked prior to transverse plane.

Continue with IBT:

2. Compare sagittal plane with coronal plane:
   a. Move the tissues in the chosen direction on a sagittal plane. Let's assume that the direction is superior again. Move the tissues in superior glide up to its limitation.
   b. While maintaining the tissues in a superior glide, now "stack on" movement of the tissues in the chosen direction on a coronal plane: clockwise or counterclockwise. Let's assume the direction is clockwise.
   c. Once the clockwise direction has been added to the superior glide, test to determine if there is greater movement then before in superior glide.

Question: Did movement in superior glide increase?

Answer:
YES. Superior glide increased. The tissue on a sagittal plane was less resistant to distortion. —*or*—
NO. Superior glide did not increase. The limitation on a sagittal plane remained the same.

Conclusion:
If the answer is YES, then coronal plane is dominant to sagittal plane.
If the answer is NO, then coronal plane is not dominant to sagittal plane. In fact, sagittal plane is dominant to coronal plane.

Application for Treatment:
If coronal plane (clockwise) is dominant to sagittal plane (superior), then coronal plane should be stacked prior to sagittal plane.
If sagittal plane is dominant to coronal plane, then sagittal plane should be stacked prior to coronal plane.

Further Testing of Other Directions:
Perform the previous steps described above, but travel in different directions (i.e. test transverse and coronal plane to determine dominance).

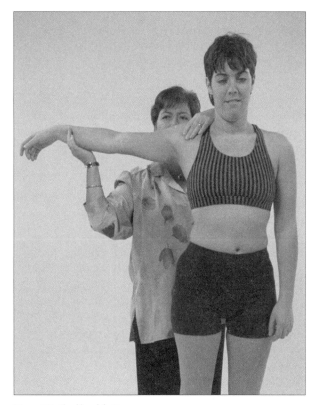

Figure 28. Shoulder abduction.

incorporate the essence of the nullification process called "Inhibitory Balance Testing and Process" into Myofascial Release. The authors thank Dr. Chauffour for his contribution to this fascial release approach.

IMPROVE ARTICULAR BALANCE
Articular balance is the maintenance of the normal relative positions of the two articular surfaces of a joint throughout full range of motion.

Articular balance—the relative positions of the two articular surfaces—should be improved after the "Release." This articular balance will be improved at hard joints and soft joints. An example of a hard joint is the glenohumeral joint, an articulation between the bony articular humerus surface, and the bony glenoid fossa. An example of a partial soft joint is the posterior surface of the soft quadriceps muscle and the bony anterior surface of the femur. An example of a total soft joint is the soft superior surface of the liver and the soft inferior surface of the diaphragm. Improved articular balance of all joints will occur with a "Release," and this should correlate with improved static posture, improved postural potential for movement, and increased physiologic ranges of motion.

Physiological Joint Movements and Accessory Joint Movements

Shoulder abduction is a physiologic movement. During abduction the humeral head glides in a caudal direction relative to the glenoid fossa.

The movement occurring at the joint surfaces of the glenohumeral joint is the accessory movement.

Example:
Soft Tissue Myofascial Release Technique of the Shoulder Girdle and Clavipectoral Fascia

INDICATION

Static postural dysfunction: Protracted shoulder girdle.

Dynamic postural dysfunction: Limitation in shoulder horizontal abduction.

POSITION

- Supine or sitting.
- One hand of the therapist is behind the scapula. The fingers are spread apart, contacting as many different tissues and structures as possible. Both *thenar eminences* can contact the humeral head. The anterior hand of the therapist rests on the *clavipectoral region.* The fingers are spread apart, again, contacting as many tissues and structures as possible. Fingers can contact *supraclavicular tissue, clavicle* and *infraclavicular tissue,* and ribs. The posterior thenar eminences contact the humeral head while the hand cups the scapula and as much tissue as the hand span allows.

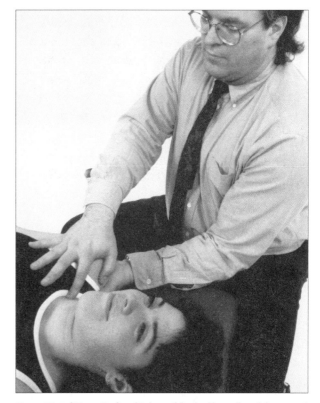

Figure 29. Soft Tissue Myofascial Release of the shoulder girdle and clavipectoral fascia.

TREATMENT

1. Compress the clavipectoral region with both hands, squeezing gently, imaging a soap bubble between the hands. Don't burst the bubble! Maintain gentle compression.

2. *First Plane:* The anterior hand moves cephalad while the posterior hand moves caudad, distorting the soap bubble. The hands return to neutral and reverse direction: the anterior hand moves the tissue caudad, while the posterior hand moves the tissue cephalad. Consider: In which directions (cephalad/caudad or caudad/cephalad) was the mobility the

greatest, and resistance least? The hands move the tissues in the indirect direction of ease, the most mobile direction. Keep hands in that new position, maintaining those directions of forces on the tissues.

3. *Second Plane:* Now add or "stack" the second plane movements. Do *not* return the hands or the tissues to neutral. Move the tissues under the anterior hand medially while the posterior hand moves the tissues laterally. Now return the tissues to neutral and compare the ease of tissue mobility when the anterior hand moves the tissues laterally while the posterior hands moves the tissues medially. Consider: Which directions (medial/lateral or lateral/medial) were the most mobile, the easiest, the least restricted? Return the tissues to that position. Maintain these directions of forces on the tissues, as well as the directions of the forces from the first plane.

4. *Third Plane:* Now add or "stack" the third plane. Do *not* return the tissues to neutral; they are displaced from neutral on two planes now. Move the tissues with the anterior hand in a clockwise direction while the posterior hand moves the tissues in a counterclockwise direction. Then return the tissues to neutral on this plane. Compare the opposite tissue distortion pattern. Move the tissues counterclockwise with the anterior hand while the posterior hand moves the tissues clockwise. Compare the two different tissue distortion patterns (clockwise/counterclockwise or counter-clockwise/clockwise. Which was the indirect pattern with the greater mobility? Return the tissues to that direction of distortion. Now there are three directions of forces from each hand onto the tissues; each hand is displacing the tissues on three planes.

5. *The Fulcrum:* Each hand exerted four different directions of forces mechanically to distort the tissue between the hands. The direction of forces were:

   • Compression
   • Superior/inferior
   • Medial/lateral
   • Clockwise/counterclockwise (medial rotation or lateral rotation).

   Each hand will now maintain all four directions of forces, maintaining a fulcrum for the tissue unwinding throughout the duration of the technique. This fulcrum will create energy, which will be transmitted into the body.

6. *The Release:* Maintain the fulcrum. As the tissue unwinds and movement occurs in the body's internal environment, there is a temptation to move the hands and release the fulcrum. *Resist the temptation to release the fulcrum.* The therapist and patient may perceive heat, paresthesia, anesthesia, vibration, fatigue, electricity, cold, perspiration, pain, circulatory changes, breathing changes, sympathetic skin erythema or blanching, and other phenomena. At the end of the technique the signs and symptoms will subside. The technique is complete when all movement, signs, symptoms, and perceptions have ceased.

RESULT

Improved postural symmetry (decreased protraction) and increased horizontal abduction.

CHAPTER 16

THE ARTICULAR MYOFASCIAL RELEASE TECHNIQUE

This chapter presents the method for and an example of "articular" or "joint" Myofascial Release. The method for and an example of the soft tissue procedure was presented in Chapter 15.

INDICATION

Articular Myofascial Release can be performed after Soft Tissue Myofascial Release. After Soft Tissue Myofascial Release is performed, residual joint dysfunction may be noted. Upon observation, static postural asymmetries may be observed at the joint. Dynamic posture evaluation may indicate positive findings of joint dysfunction: lack of articular balance. Mobility testing will confirm joint hypomobility. Articular Myofascial Release will affect joint capsule and ligaments.

GENERAL GUIDELINE: APPLY THE 3-PLANAR CONCEPT
3-Planar Fascial Fulcrum techniques access the body on three planes: sagittal, coronal, and transverse.

TREATMENT

1. Place your hands on either side of the joint. Hold the bones close to the two articular surfaces. (Occasionally a longer lever is more feasible). Grip only as hard as is necessary to maintain control of the position of both joint surfaces. Do not distract or approximate the joint surfaces. Move your hands in opposite directions on all three planes (sagittal, coronal, transverse). On the sagittal plane, move one joint surface superior while the other joint surface is moved inferior (superior/inferior). Then move the joint surface in the opposite direction (inferior/superior). On a transverse plane, move one joint surface into medial rotation while the other is moved in the direction of a lateral (medial/lateral) rotation. Then change directions of movement of the joint surfaces (lateral/medial). On a coronal plane, move one joint surface in an abduction direction, while the other is move in an adduction direction. Then change the directions of movement of joint surfaces. Move indirectly in the direction of ease (greatest joint mobility). Stack these accessory and "joint play" movements.

2. *The Fulcrum:* Maintain your grip on the body parts and maintain the direction of force on the three planes that you initiated to displace the joint surfaces. This is your fulcrum around which the fascial tissues (ligaments, capsule) surrounding the joint will unwind.

3. *The Release:* Maintain the fulcrum. Do not move your hands with the tissue movement. *Resist the temptation.* Allow for repositioning of joint surfaces during the technique for improved articular balance. Fascial unwinding will be slow and gentle. Near the completion of the treatment, there may be a "clunking" or other joint "noises" as a result of the rebalancing of joint surfaces. At the end of the release your hands will be in a neutral position, and articular balance will be improved.

RESULT

Normalization of articular balance and improved joint mobility.

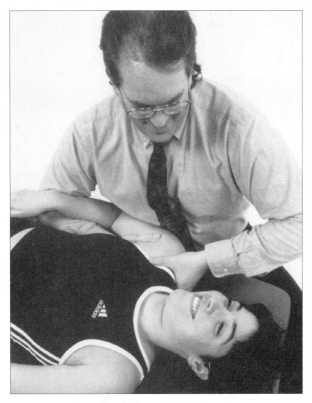

Figure 30. Articular Myofascial Release of the glenohumeral joint.

Articular Fulcrum Myofascial Release Technique of the Glenohumeral Joint

INDICATION

Static postural dysfunction; for example, anterior shear of the humeral head in the glenoid fossa. Dynamic postural dysfunction; for example, limitation in some end ranges of shoulder motions, with hypomobility of accessory joint movements evident on mobility testing.

POSITION

- Supine or sitting.
- One hand of the therapist grips the shoulder girdle to control the position of the glenoid fossa. The other hand grips the upper arm to control the position of the humeral head. *Do not distract or approximate the joint surface.*

TREATMENT

1. *First Plane:* The superior hand on the shoulder girdle lifts the glenoid fossa cephalad, while the inferior hand on the upper arm pulls the humeral head caudad; then return the joint surfaces to neutral and reverse the directions of the articular surfaces. The superior hand pushes the glenoid fossa caudad, while the inferior hand pushes the humeral head cephalad. Consider: Which direction (cephalad/ caudad or caudad/cephalad) was the most mobile, the least restricted, and the least inhibited? Return the joint surfaces to the position of greatest mobility. Maintain the position of the articular surface on this plane.

2. *Second Plane:* Now add or "stack" the second plane movements. The superior hand holding the shoulder girdle can push the glenoid fossa anteriorly while the inferior hand, holding the upper arm, can

push the humeral head posteriorly; then return the joint surfaces to neutral and reverse the directions of the articular surfaces. The superior hand now pushes the glenoid fossa posteriorly, while the inferior hand pushes the humeral head anteriorly. Compare the directions (anterior/posterior or posterior/anterior). Move the joint surface in the indirect directions of ease. Maintain the articular surface in this new position. Now each articular surface is displaced in two different directions.

3. *Third Plane:* Now add or "stack" the third plane movements. The superior hand gripping the shoulder girdle can rotate the glenoid fossa externally while the inferior hand, gripping the upper arm, rotates the humeral head internally; then return the joint surfaces to neutral and reverse the directions. The superior hand can push the glenoid fossa into internal rotation, while the inferior hand moves the humeral head into external rotation. Compare the directions (external/internal rotations or internal/external rotations). Move the articular surfaces on this plane in the indirect direction of greatest mobility. Maintain the positions of the articular surfaces on this plane. Now the three directions of forces asserted to displace each articluar surface are maintained.

4. *The Fulcrum:* Each hand has exerted three different directions of forces to mechanically move and position the articular surfaces in opposite directions on three planes. Each hand will now maintain all three directions of forces, maintaining a fulcrum for the tissue unwinding of joint capsule and ligaments throughout the duration of the technique.

5. *The Release:* Maintain the fulcrum. As the tissue unwinds and sensations of extra-cellular and intra-cellular movement are perceived, there is a temptation to move the hands and release the fulcrum. Resist the temptation to release the fulcrum. Maintain the fulcrum until all movement, all signs, all symptoms, and all perceptions have ceased.

RESULT

Improved articular balance. Normal articular balance of humeral head within the glenoid fossa; increased joint mobility; increased ranges of motion.

CHAPTER 17

THE SPINAL SYSTEM

Mobilization of Spine: The Pelvic Joints

Basic Concepts of Specific Articular Release Techniques

- Hands move in opposite directions
- 3-Planar concept
- There is no compression and no distraction of the joint surfaces
- Grasp at both ends of the joint, as close to the joint as possible
- Move the (bony) articular surfaces
- Accessory and "joint play" movements are affected
- Indirect direction of ease
- Fulcrum
- Maintain the fulcrum until "The Release."

Anterior Iliosacral Joint Release

INDICATION

This technique affects pelvic mobility, sitting balance, and standing balance. This technique is effective with recurrent biomechanical dysfunction of pubic symphysis and iliosacral joint. Trunk elongation is improved. Soft tissue dysfunction in the pelvic bowl is affected.

POSITION

- Supine.
- Therapist stands facing the feet of the patient with back to the patient's head.
- Hands cup the bilateral ilia. The thumbs are medial to the *anterior superior iliac spine (ASIS)*. The fingers are spread apart, wrapping lightly around the lateral aspect of the pelvis. Image that the sacrum has been "removed" and that one joint surface of the ilium is moving against the other joint surface of the second ilium.

TREATMENT

1. *First* and *Second Planes:* Move the right ilium posterior and medial. Move the left ilium anterior and lateral; then, change directions. Move the right ilium anterior and lateral while the left ilium is moved posterior and medial. Assess the most mobile pattern of pelvic movement. Move the ilia in the directions of ease (posterio-medial/ anterolateral or anterolateral/ poseromedial).

2. *Third Plane:* Now add or "stack" the third plane movement. Move the right ilium

superior and the left ilium inferior; then change directions, moving the right ilium inferior while the left ilium is being moved superior. Move the ilia in the direction of ease (superior/inferior or inferior/superior).

3. *The Fulcrum:* Maintain your grip on the body parts and maintain the direction of force on the three planes that you initiated to displace the joint surfaces. This is your fulcrum around which the fascial tissues (ligaments, capsule) surrounding the joint will unwind.

4. *The Release:* Maintain the fulcrum. Do not move your hands with the tissue movement. *Resist the temptation.* Allow for repositioning of joint surfaces during the technique for improved articular balance. Fascial unwinding will be slow and gentle. Near the completion of the treatment, there may be a "clunking" or other joint "noises" as a result of the rebalancing of joint surfaces. At the end of the release your hands will be in a neutral position, and articular balance will be improved.

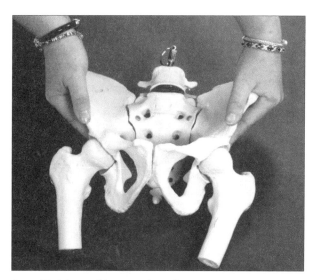

Figure 31. Palpation of the anterior iliosacral joint.

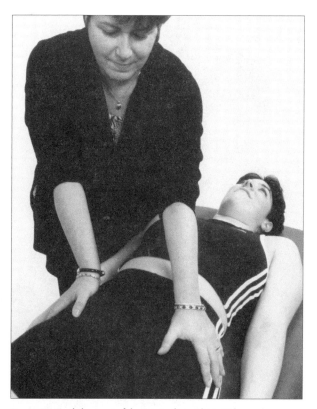

Figure 32. Hand placements of the Anterior Iliosacral Joint Release.

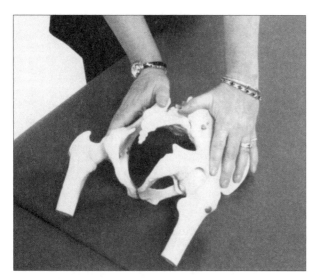

Figure 33. Palpation of the posterior iliosacral joint.

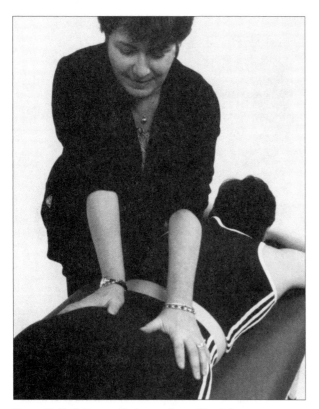

Figure 34. Hand placements for Posterior Iliosacral Joint Release.

Posterior Iliosacral Joint Release

INDICATION

This technique is effective for all low back pain. Pelvic stability, balance, standing, and ambulation are improved with this technique.

POSITION

- Prone.
- The therapist stands facing the patient's feet with back to the client's head.
- Therapist's hands grip the ilia (buttocks). Place the thumb lateral to the sacroliliac joint line. Image that the sacrum has been removed and that the joint surfaces on the ilia articulate with each other.

TREATMENT

1. *First* and *Second Planes:* Move the right ilium anterior and lateral; move the left ilium posterior and medial; then change directions: move the right ilium posterior and medial while the left ilium is moved anterior and lateral. Assess the direction of ease. Move the ilia in the indirect direction of least restriction.

2. *Third Plane:* Now add or "stack" the third plane movements. Move the right ilium superior and the left inferior; then change directions: move the right ilium inferior while the left ilium is moved superior. Move the ilia in three directions of ease on three planes.

3. *The Fulcrum:* Maintain your grip on the body parts and maintain the direction of force on the three planes that you initiated to displace the joint surfaces. This is your fulcrum around which the fascial tissues (ligaments, capsule) surrounding the joint will unwind.

4. *The Release:* Maintain the fulcrum. Do not move your hands with the tissue movement. *Resist the temptation.* Allow for repositioning of joint surfaces during the technique for improved articular balance. Fascial unwinding will be slow and gentle. Near the completion of the treatment, there may be a "clunking" or other joint "noises" as a result of the rebalancing of joint surfaces. At the end of the release your hands will be in a neutral position, and articular balance will be improved.

The Sacrum Release

The sacrum is the most crucial structure to be mobilized. The dura mater attaches at S2 at the *sacrococcygal joint,* and at the *coccyx.* Via mobilization of sacrum, restrictions of the dura mater and spinal cord will be affected.

INDICATION

This technique is especially indicated for all patients to release the dura mater attachment at S2 and to release impingement of sacral plexus nerves. Chronic sacroiliac joint dysfunction responds well. This technique is essential for all orthopedic, neurologic, pediatric, and geriatric patients.

POSITION

- Prone.
- The therapist stands facing the client's feet with back to the patient's head.
- Place thenar eminences and thumbs on the sacrum along the length of the lateral margins, just medial to the sacroiliac joint lines. Thumbs and thenar eminences control the position of the joint surfaces of sacrum. Image that the sacrum is in two halves, a right and left side.

TREATMENT

1. *First Plane:* Move the right articular surface of sacrum superior and the left articular surface inferior; then change direction of forces and move the right sacral joint surface inferior while the left sacral joint is moved superior. Assess the direction of ease. Move the sacrum in the indirect direction of least resistance.

2. *Second Plane:* Now add or "stack" the second plane movements. Move the right sacral articular surface anterior. The left rests without pressure. Then push the left sacral articular surface anterior, while the

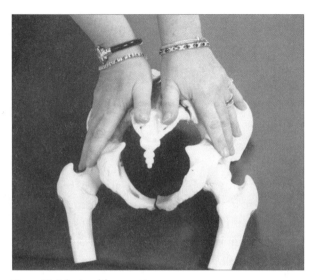

Figure 35. Palpation of the sacrum in prone.

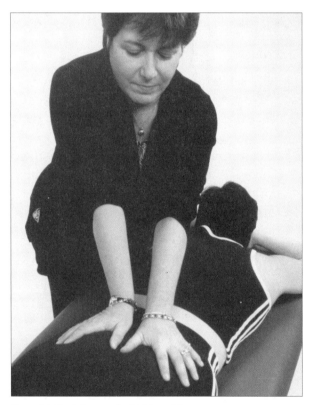

Figure 36. Hand placement for the Sacrum Release.

right rests without pressure. Assess and move the sacrum in the direction of ease.

3. *Third Plane:* Now add or "stack" the third plane movement. Move the right sacral articular surface in anterior rotation, the left in posterior rotation. Then change the directions of forces and move the right sacral articular surface in posterior rotation while the left sacral articular surface is moved in anterior rotation. Assess and move sacrum in the direction of ease.

4. *The Fulcrum:* Maintain your grip on the body parts and maintain the direction of force on the three planes that you initiated to displace the joint surfaces. This is your fulcrum around which the fascial tissues (ligaments, capsule) surrounding the joint will unwind.

5. *The Release:* Maintain the fulcrum. Do not move your hands with the tissue movement. *Resist the temptation.* Allow for repositioning of joint surfaces during the technique for improved articular balance. Fascial unwinding will be slow and gentle. Near the completion of the treatment, there may be a "clunking" or other joint "noises" as a result of the rebalancing of joint surfaces. At the end of the release your hands will be in a neutral position, and articular balance will be improved.

The Lumbrosacral Junction Release

INDICATION

This technique is very effective for increasing reciprocal mobility of L5/S1. Reciprocal gait is affected. It is essential for all low back pain patients, especially patients with a history of discopathy.

POSITION

- Prone.
- Place one thumb and thenar eminence on L5. Place the other thumb and thenar eminence on the sacral base. Thumbs are very close together.

TREATMENT

1. *First Plane:* Move L5 to the right and move sacral base to the left; then change directions of forces and move L5 to the left and sacral base to the right. Assess and move in the directions of least restrictions.

2. *Second Plane:* Now add or "stack" the second plane movements. Move L5 into right rotation and move sacral base into left rotation; then change direction of forces and move L5 into left rotation and sacral base into right rotation. Assess and move in the directions of least restrictions.

3. *Third Plane:* Now add or "stack" the third plane movements. Move L5 into right sidebending and move sacral base into left sidebending; then change directions of forces and move L5 into left sidebending and move sacral base into right sidebending. Assess and move in the directions of least restrictions.

2. *The Fulcrum:* Maintain your grip on the body parts and maintain the direction of force on the three planes that you initiated to displace the joint surfaces. This is your fulcrum around which the fascial tissues

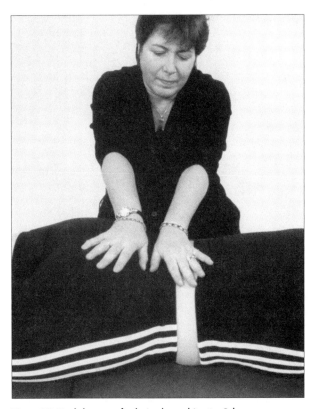

Figure 37. Hand placements for the Lumbosacral Junction Release.

(ligaments, capsule) surrounding the joint will unwind.

3. *The Release:* Maintain the fulcrum. Do not move your hands with the tissue movement. *Resist the temptation.* Allow for repositioning of joint surfaces during the technique for improved articular balance. Fascial unwinding will be slow and gentle. Near the completion of the treatment, there may be a "clunking" or other joint "noises" as a result of the rebalancing of joint surfaces. At the end of the release your hands will be in a neutral position, and articular balance will be improved.

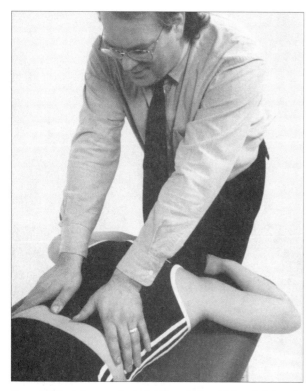

Figure 38. Hand placements for the Soft Tissue Myofascial Release Technique of the thoracolumbar junction.

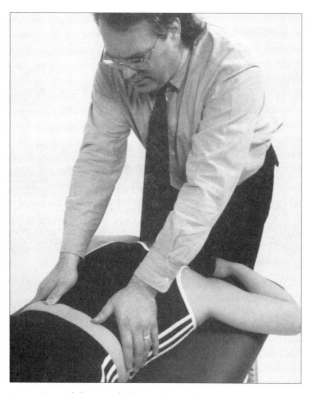

Figure 39. Hand placements for the Articular Myofascial Release Technique of the thoracolumbar junction.

The Thoracolumbar Junction Release

INDICATION

This technique is excellent to improve respiratory status, trunk control, and trunk mobility.

Phase 1: Specific Soft Tissue Myofasical Release Technique for the Thoracolumbar Junction

POSITION

- Prone.
- The therapist stands facing the patient's feet.
- The head is midline.
- Place thumbs on either side of the *thoracolumbar junction,* a few inches apart. Fingers are spread out. Fingers lie along the length of the ribs.

TREATMENT

1. *First Plane:* Move right hand superior, the left hand inferior; then change directions of forces and move the right hand inferior and the left hand superior. Assess and move in the direction of least restrictions.

2. *Second Plane:* Now add or "stack" the second plane movement. Move both hands together with rotation clockwise; then both hands together, rotation counterclockwise. Assess and move in the direction of least restriction. Note that in this plane, the hands are not moving in opposite directions.

3. *Tissue Tension Release:* Maintain the fulcrum. The hands do not move. They do not follow the tissue movements, although the temptation to move the hands and follow the tissue motion will be great. The goal is not a physiologic unwinding of a body part. The objective is the internal "unraveling" of the fascial tissue. By

maintaining the fulcrum, energy will be created/transduced. The force of the energy causing the fascial release will produce more changes in the internal environment of the connective tissue. The fascial unwinding will be slow and gentle. Do not allow quick or repetitive or forceful physiologic movements.

Phase 2: Specific Articular Myofascial Release Technique for Thoracolumbar Junction

POSITION

- Prone.
- The head is midline.
- Place thumbs on either side of the thoracolumbar junction, a few inches apart. The hands "take up the slack" of the soft tissue and the *fingers grip the ribs*. This technique mobilizes the bony rib structures.

TREATMENT

1. *First Plane:* The right hand moves ribs cephalad while the left hand moves ribs caudad; then change directions and the right hand moves ribs caudad while the left hand moves ribs cephalad. Assess and move in the direction of least restrictions.

2. *Second Plane:* Now add or "stack" the second plane movement. The right hand moves ribs anterior; the left hand move ribs anterior. Assess and move in directions of least restriction.

3. *Third Plane:* Now add or "stack" the third plane movement. The right hand moves ribs into anterior rotation while the left hand moves ribs into posterior rotation; then change directions and the right hand moves ribs into posterior rotation while the left hand moves ribs into anterior rotation. Assess and move in the directions of least restrictions.

4. *The Fulcrum:* Maintain your grip on the body parts and maintain the direction of force on the three planes that you initiated to displace the joint surfaces. This is your fulcrum around which the fascial tissues (ligaments, capsule) surrounding the joint will unwind.

5. *The Release:* Maintain the fulcrum. Do not move your hands with the tissue movement. *Resist the temptation.* Allow for repositioning of joint surfaces during the technique for improved articular balance. Fascial unwinding will be slow and gentle. Near the completion of the treatment, there may be a "clunking" or other joint "noises" as a result of the rebalancing of joint surfaces. At the end of the release your hands will be in a neutral position, and articular balance will be improved.

The Facilitated Segment and the Facilitated Spine

By "facilitated segment" is meant the hyperactivity of the myotatic reflex arc at a given vertebral segment, including increased *gamma gain*, *afferent gain*, and *efferent gain*. The excessive and high frequency discharge from sensory input due to neuromusculoskeletal dysfunction is distributed throughout the central nervous system. This results in hyperactivity of the spinal cord. *De-facilitation* of the spine is a generic technique to decrease the excessive and high frequency discharge through the spinal cord.

De-facilitation of the Spine

INDICATION

This technique is effective in attaining a general decrease in hypertonicity.

POSITION

- Supine.
- The therapist stands at the side of the patient, facing the head. One hand lies between straight legs; the sacrum rests on the palm of that hand. The therapist leans on their elbow in order to avoid exciting a torque force on the sacrum. Fingers lie flat, not curled into L5/S1.

TREATMENT

1. While palm remains under sacrum, gently compress up the spine one segment at a time: L5/S1, L5/L4, L4/L3, and so on. The amount of forced exerted is *less than 5 grams* (the weight of a nickel). The *intention* to compress is important. The therapist can attempt to "visualize" how far up the spine the compression force is progressing. If a "barrier" is encountered (a tissue resistance), release the compression slightly just "before" the barrier. Inserting two fingers of the other hand beneath the spine and "contacting" the segment of the barrier can facilitate a release past the barrier. After the release of the barrier, continue to compress up the spine until occiput is reached.

2. *The Fulcrum:* Maintain the 5 grams of compression force until the "de-facilitation" process has occurred up to the Craniocervical junction.

3. *The Release:* Maintain the fulcrum. Do not "follow" the movement of the sacrum. Maintain the fulcrum cephalad on sacrum with 5 grams of force until all perception of movement, signs, symptoms and tissue tension changes have ceased for therapist and patient. A distraction force by the body will follow. Allow the spine to elongate.

The following photos are a progression of steps. They illustrate how to place the practitioner's hand under the sacrum (between the legs of the patient) in a 'non-invasive manner' to perform the De-facilitation of the Spine at Sacrum. Please instruct the patient accordingly with the following steps.

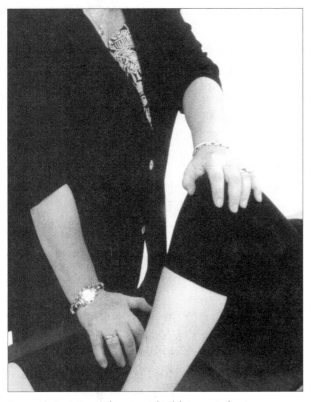

Figure 40. Step1: Instruct the patient to bend their opposite knee.

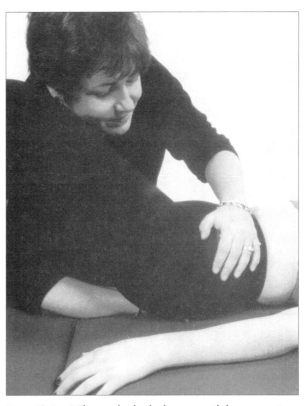

Figure 42. Step 3: Place your hand under their sacrum with the sacrum resting comfortably in the palm of your hand.

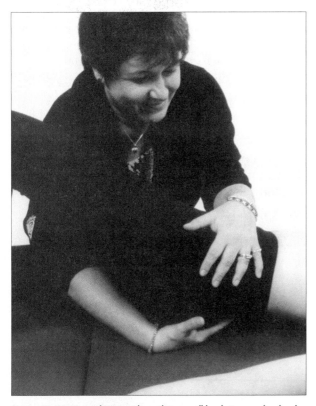

Figure 41. Step 2: Let the patient know that you will be placing your hand under their sacrum. Instruct the patient to roll their pelvis off the table on the opposite side.

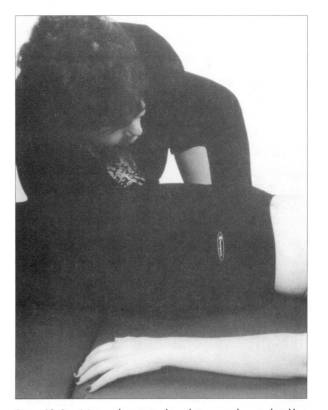

Figure 43. Step 4: Instruct the patient to lower their opposite leg onto the table and relax on your hand. Rest your own forearm and elbow on the table between the legs of the patient.

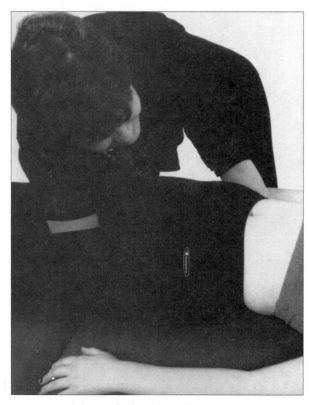

Figure 44. Hand placement for the Lumbosacral Decompression Technique.

Myofascial Release of the Lumbarsacral Junction and Nerve Root Impingements

Phase 1: Lumbosacral Decompression

Lumbosacral decompression is essential for all patients. The *craniocervical junction* cannot be completely mobilized with the compression of L5/S1.

POSITION

- Supine.
- The position of this technique is the same as the De-facilitation of the Spine Technique. One hand inserts between straight legs; the sacrum rests on the palm of that hand. The therapist leans on her elbow in order to avoid exciting a torque force on the sacrum. Fingers lie flat, not curled into L5/S1. The other hand inserts under the low back to fixate L5 spinous process.

TREATMENT

1. Gently, with 5 grams of force (the weight of a nickel), distract the sacrum caudad towards the feet, with intent to distract the lumbosacral junction. As the tissue at the lumbosacral junction releases, distraction will occur between L5 and S1.
2. *The Fulcrum:* Do not "follow" sacrum. Maintain the longitudinal direction of distraction with 5 grams of force.
3. *The Release:* Maintain the fulcrum caudad on sacrum with 5 grams of force until all perception of movement, signs, symptoms and tissue tension changes have ceased for therapist and patient. The fascial unwinding will be slow and gentle.

Phase 2: Release of Extradural Impingements from Lumbosacral Decompression

INDICATION

Indicated with all nerve root impingements, e.g., sciatica.

TREATMENT

1. Maintain the lumbosacral decompression of Phase 1 until the release is complete.

2. Once the release is complete, remove the hand that is fixating L5 from beneath the low back. Continue to distract sacrum gently, one segment at a time: L5/L4, L4/L3, L3/L2, and so on, until occiput is reached.

3. If a "barrier" is encountered (an obstacle to further release), release the distraction force slightly until just before the barrier. Inserting two fingers of the other hand beneath the spine and contacting the barrier segment can facilitate release of the barrier. (See Figure 44.)

4. *The Release:* Maintain the fulcrum with 5 grams of force until all perception of movement, signs, symptoms and tissue tension changes have ceased for therapist and patient. The fascial unwinding will be slow and gentle.

Craniocervical Junction: A Specific Myofascial Release Technique

INDICATION

Nerve root impingement, e.g., cervical syndrome.

To decompress subocciptal space in TMJ and craniofacial patients.

To decompress the subocciptal space when there is a compromise of: the spinal accessory nerve, causing torticollis or trapezius spasm; the glosso-pharyngeal nerve and hypoglossal nerve, causing tongue thrust and other swallowing dysfunction, sinus congestion; and the vagus nerve for hyper-activity in children.

POSITION

- Supine.
- The therapist sits at the head of the patient.
- Finger positions change through treatment

Phase 1: Craniocervical Release

TREATMENT

1. Place the third finger of each hand, one on top of the other, under the head. Rest the head at the *inion* (at the middle of the *superior nuchal line* of the occiput, external to the *confluence of sinuses*), on the pad of the *distal phalanx* of the top third finger. (See Figures 46 to 48.)

2. Maintain the head as in Step 1, in a resting position, until there is a "softening." Do not put any force on the head. Maintain a relaxed hand and third finger under inion.

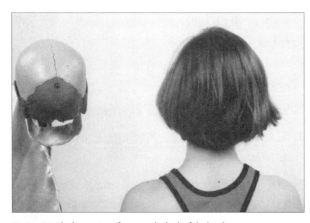

Figure 45. The locomotion of inion at the back of the head.

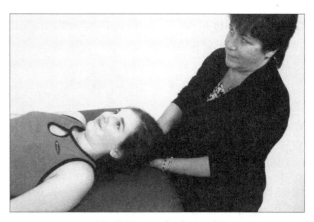

Figure 48. Position with hand placements for Phase 1 of the Craniocervical Release.

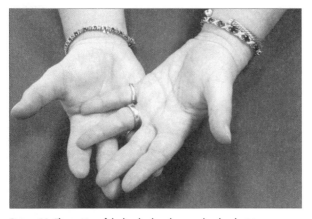

Figure 46. The position of the hands when they are placed under inion.

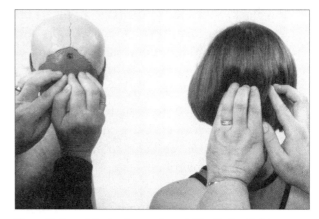

Figure 49. Anatomic landmark at superior nuchal line (for Step 3 of the Craniocervical Release).

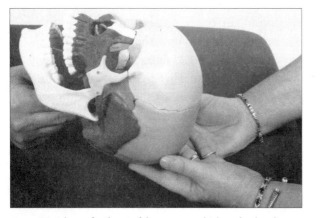

Figure 47. Palpation for Phase 1 of the Craniocervical Release, hands under inion.

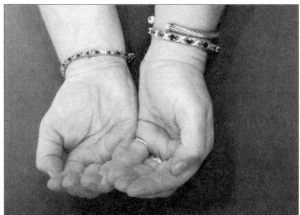

Figure 50. Hand position for Step 3 of the Craniocervical Release, the "soldier" position.

3. Hold the fingers together in an upright fashion like "soldiers" with 90 degrees of flexion at the *metacarpalphalangeal joints* and full extension at the *interphalangeal joints*. Rest the head at the superior nuchal line, external to the transverse sinus, on the tips of the fingers. Maintain the head thus, until there is a "softening." Do not exert any force on the head.

4. Maintain the "soldier" position with the fingers. Visualize that there is a laterally directed force spreading the hands gently apart until a lateral "spreading" at the transverse sinus is felt. Use only 5 grams of force; intent is important. Do not really move the hands.

5. Maintain the fingers again in a "soldier" position. Move the fingers to rest just caudal to occiput. Maintain minimal pressure superior against the occiput. The suboccipital space is resting on the tips of the fingers. The fingers will gradually sink anteriorly between the *arch of atlas* and the occiput. Maintain this position until there is a complete "softening."

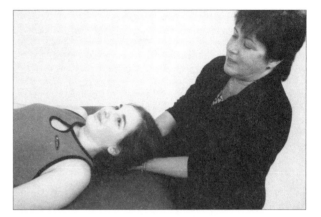

Figure 51. Hand placements and patient position for Step 3 of the Craniocervical Release.

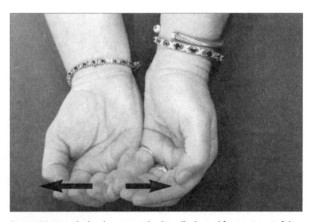

Figure 52. View the hand position with a laterally directed force in Step 4 of the Craniocervical Release.

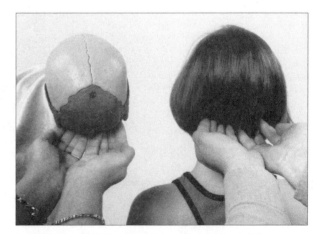

Figure 53. Anatomic landmark for sub-occipital space in Step 5 of the Craniocervical Release.

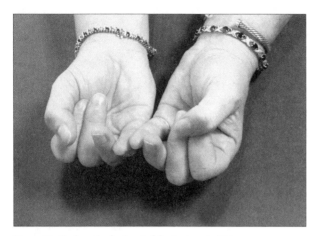

Figure 54. Hand position for Step 6 of the Craniocervical Release.

6. Maintain the same finger position. With the distal phalanxes of the fourth and fifth fingers of both hands, press them cephalad against the occiput. Maintain, at most, 5 grams of force superiorly with those fourth and fifth fingers, while the other fingers maintain the space between occiput and atlas. Continue with this minimal pressure until there is no further "release." The subocciptal space will be more open.

Phase 2: Release of Extradural Impingement from Craniocervical Region

TREATMENT

1. Once the occiput is released from the atlas, maintain the "soldiers" position of the fingers. With 5 grams of force, distract down the kinetic chain one segment at a time: C1/C2, C2/C3, C3/C4, etc.

2. If a "barrier" is encountered, release the distraction force until just before the barrier.

3. Distract to the end of the dura mater insertion on coccyx.

5. Visualize where the distraction force is, as the force of the technique progresses down the spine. Maintain the 5 grams of force until there is no further "release."

Fascial Release Technique to Balance the Cranial Dura

APPLICATION

Thoracic inlet transverse process must be released prior to these techniques.

INDICATION

This technique is gentle and effectively balances the falx cerebri, falx cerebellum, and tentorium cerebellum.

Phase 1: Lateral Vault Hold

POSITION

- Supine.
- The therapist sits at the head of the table holding the patient's head with palms of hands over the parietal and temporal regions. The temporoparietal suture should be in the palm of the hand, with fingers spread out.

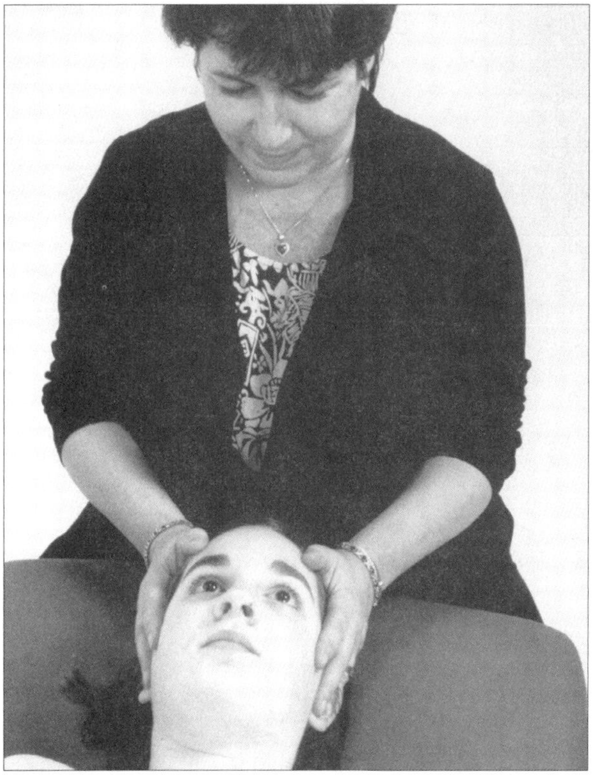

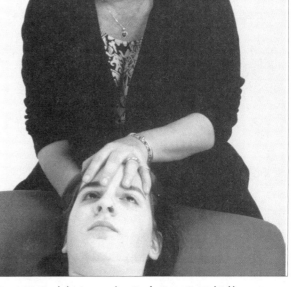

Figure 55. Hand placements and position for the Lateral Vault Hold.

TREATMENT

1. Compress hand medially with a force of no more than 5 grams (not enough force to burst a soap bubble). Maintain this compression force.

2. Hands rotate in opposite directions: anterior and posterior rotation on a sagittal plane. Move the tissue indirectly. *If, as a therapist you are not skilled in cranial therapies, proceed with care: utilize "intent" and mobilize the tissue only a few degrees. Do not go to the end of available mobility.*

3. *The Release:* Maintain the fulcrum. Wait for a completed release. Release is complete when all perception of movement, signs, symptoms, and tissue tension changes have ceased.

Figure 56. Hand placements and position for Fronto-Occipital Hold.

Phase 2: Fronto-Occipital Hold

POSITION

- Supine.
- The therapist sits at patient's head.
- The occiput rests on the palm of the bottom hand. The top hand rests, spread out, and palm down, on the frontal. Fingertips extend over the eyebrows.

TREATMENT

1. Compress hand with a force of no more than 5 grams (not enough to burst a soap bubble). Maintain this compression force.

2. Hands move in opposite directions: clockwise and counterclockwise rotations on a coronal plane. Go Indirect. *If, as a therapist you are not skilled in cranial therapies, proceed with care: utilize "intent" and mobilize the tissue only a few degrees. Do not go to the end of available mobility.*

3. *The Release:* Maintain the fulcrum. Wait for a completed release. Release is complete when all perception of movement, signs, symptoms, and tissue tension changes have ceased.

CHAPTER 18

SPECIALIZED MYOFASCIAL RELEASE TECHNIQUES

Muscle Belly Technique

INDICATION

This technique is appropriate for quadriceps, hamstrings, gastrocnemius, tibialis anterior, deltoid, biceps, and brachioradialis.

POSITION

- Place both hands, side by side, on the muscle belly.

TREATMENT

1. Grip the mucle belly gently but firmly. Move the muscle in three directions (on three planes). Go Indirect.

2. *First Plane:* Move the muscle superior and inferior. Move in the direction of ease.

3. *Second Plane:* Now add or "stack" the second plane movements. Move the muscle medial and lateral. Move in the direction of ease.

4. *Third Plane:* Now add or "stack" the third plane. Move the muscle clockwise and counterclockwise. Move in the direction of ease.

5. *The Release:* Maintain the fulcrum created in Steps 1 to 4. As the tissue unwinds and movement occurs in the body's internal environment, there is a temptation to move the hands and release the fulcrum. *Resist the temptation to release the fulcrum.*

Note: This technique is like a modified Articular Myofascial Release: soft tissue articulating with bone.

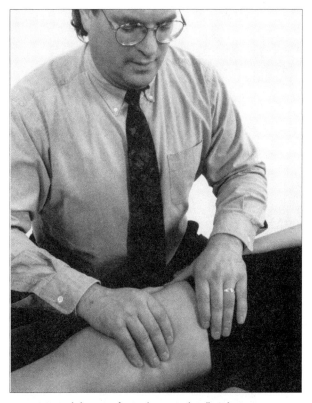

Figure 57. Hand placements for Quadriceps Muscle Belly Technique.

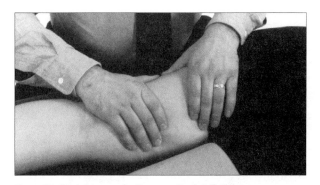

Figure 58. Hand placements for Hamstrings Muscle Belly Technique.

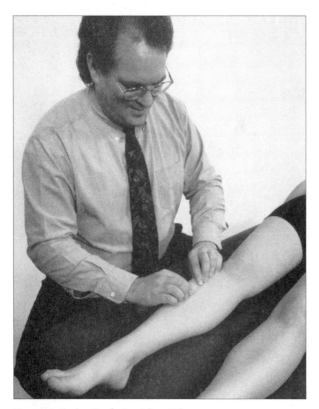

Figure 59. Hand position for Scar Release Technique.

Scar Tissue Release

INDICATION

This technique can address all scar tissue.

APPLICATION

This technique should be performed after an application of a general Soft Tissue Myofascial Release has been preformed over the area.

POSITION

- Place the pads of the distal phalanxes of the fingers of one or both hands along the length of the scar. If the scar is very small, use two or three fingers.

TREATMENT

1. Press firmly on the scar tissue and maintain the pressure. Each successive repetition will require greater compression to "take up the slack" of the soft tissue. Be tissue specific for the scar tissue. Move the scar in three directions (on three planes). Go Indirect.

2. *First Plane:* Move the scar superior and inferior. Move in the direction of ease.

3. *Second Plane:* Now add or "stack" the second plane movements. Move the scar medial and lateral. Move in the direction of ease.

4. *Third Plane:* Now add or "stack" the third plane. Move the scar clockwise and counterclockwise. Move in the direction of ease.

5. *The Release:* Maintain the fulcrum created in Steps 1 to 4. As the tissue unwinds and movement occurs in the body's internal environment, there is a temptation to move the hands and release the fulcrum. *Resist the temptation to release the fulcrum.*

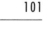

Capsule, Ligament, Tendon, and Retinaculum Release

INDICATION

This technique is very effective in increasing soft tissue mobility of the more chronic and deep fascial restrictions in dysfunction including: carpal tunnel, anterior compartment of arm and leg, supraspinatus, bicipital tendonitis, epicondylitis, DeQuervains, medial and lateral ligaments of knee, tarsal tunnel and plantar fascitis.

APPLICATION

These specific techniques are performed after an application of a general Soft Tissue Myofascial Release.

POSITION

- "Sandwich" the wrist. Use direct finger pad contact. Be site and tissue specific.

TREATMENT

1. Compress gently but firmly until there is palpation of specific tissue (e.g., ligament). Maintain finger pressure to affect the deeper tissue (i.e., the *carpal retinaculum*). Move either the capsule, ligament, tendon, or retinaculum in three directions (on three planes). Go indirect.

2. *First Plane:* Move the capsule, ligament, tendon, or retinaculum superior and inferior. Move in the direction of ease.

3. *Second Plane:* Now add or "stack" the second plane movements. Move the capsule, ligament, tendon, or retinaculum medial and lateral. Move in the direction of ease.

4. *Third Plane:* Now add or "stack" the third plane. Move the capsule, ligament, tendon, or retinaculum clockwise and counter-clockwise. Move in the direction of ease.

Figure 60. Hand position for Capsule Release at the glenohumeral joint capsule.

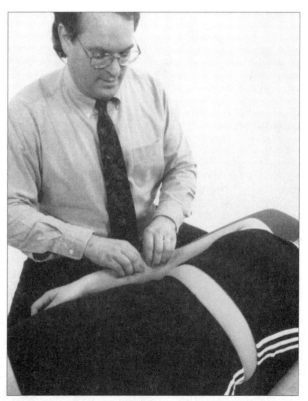

Figure 61. Hand position for Ligament Release at the proximal radial head ligament.

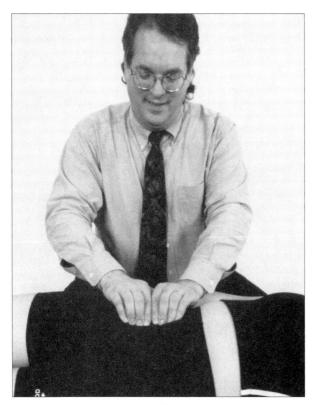

Figure 62. Hand position for Ligament Release at the inguinal ligament.

5. *The Release:* Maintain the fulcrum created in Steps 1 to 4. As the tissue unwinds and movement occurs in the body's internal environment, there is a temptation to move the hands and release the fulcrum. *Resist the temptation to release the fulcrum.*

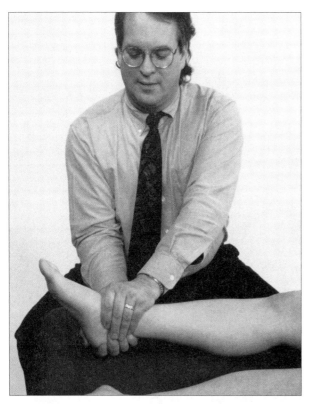

Figure 63. Hand position for Retinaculum Release at the tarsal tunnel.

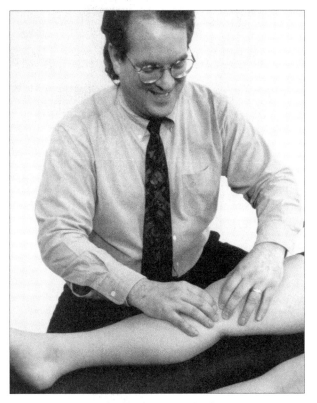

Figure 64. Hand position for the Knee Joint Capsule Release.

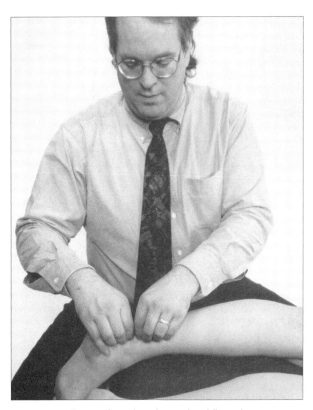

Figure 66. Hand position for Tendon Release at the Achilles tendon.

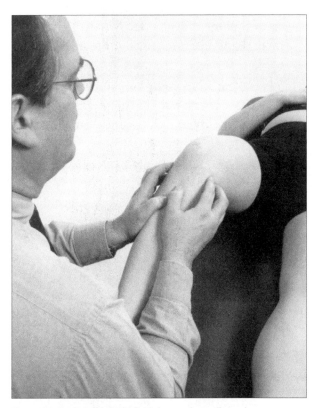

Figure 65. Hand position for Tendon Release at the patellar tendon.

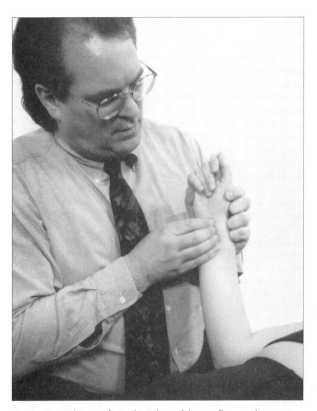

Figure 67. Hand position for Tendon Release of the wrist flexor tendons.

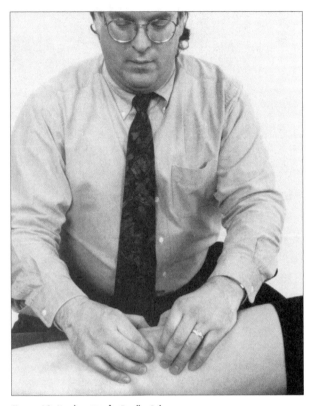

Figure 68. Hand position for Patellar Release.

Patellar Release

INDICATION

Chondromalacia: recurrent patellar dislocation.

APPLICATION

This technique is performed after an application of a general Soft Tissue Myofascial Release and a general Articular Myofascial Release to the knee. It can be performed after an application of Muscle Belly technique for the quadriceps.

POSITION

- Grip patella with fingers of both hands.

TREATMENT

1. Move the patella in three directions (on three planes). Go indirect.
2. *First Plane:* Move the patella superior and inferior. Move in the direction of ease.
3. *Second Plane:* Now add or "stack" the second plane movements. Move the patella medial and lateral. Move in the direction of ease.
4. *Third Plane:* Now add or "stack" the third plane. Move the patella clockwise and counterclockwise. Move in the direction of ease.
5. *The Release:* Maintain the fulcrum created in Steps 1 to 4. As the tissue unwinds and movement occurs in the body's internal environment, there is a temptation to move the hands and release the fulcrum. *Resist the temptation to release the fulcrum.*

Hyoid System

INDICATION

This technique is effective for all swallowing and articulation dysfunctions, for example, with temporo-mandibular joint dysfunction (TMJ). It is essential for treatment of neurologic patients which chronic scar tissue post tracheotomy.

POSITION: PHASE ONE

- Supine.
- The therapist sits facing the side of the patient.
- The occiput rests in the therapist's superior hand. Thumb and index finger of caudal hand gently grip the angles of mandible.

TREATMENT: PHASE ONE

1. *First Plane:* Move occiput and mandible in opposite directions: medial/lateral. Move in the direction of ease.

2. *Second Plane:* Now add or "stack" the second plane movements. Move occiput and mandible in opposite directions: anterior/posterior. Move in the direction of ease.

3. *Third Plane:* Now add or "stack" the third plane. Move occiput and mandible in opposite directions: right/left rotation (clockwise/counterclockwise). Move in the direction of ease.

4. *The Release:* Maintain the fulcrum created in Steps 1 to 4. As the tissue unwinds and movement occurs in the body's internal environment, there is a temptation to move the hands and release the fulcrum. *Resist the temptation to release the fulcrum.*

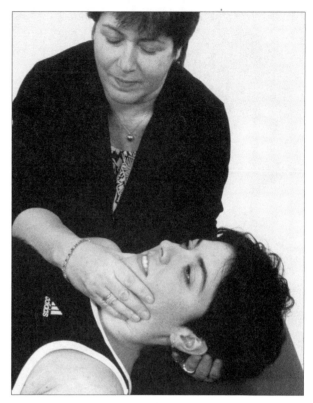

Figure 69. Hand position for Phase 1 of the Hyoid Release.

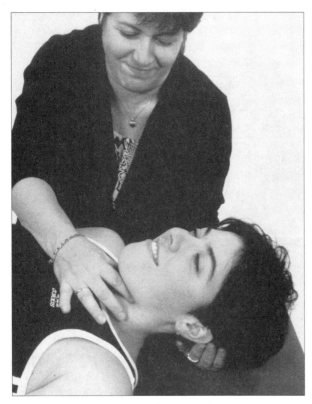

Figure 70. Hand position for Phase 2 of the Hyoid Release.

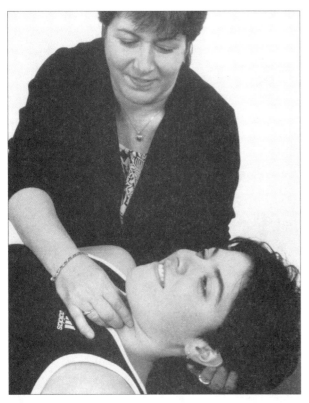

Figure 71. Hand position for Phase 3 of the Hyoid Release.

POSITION: PHASE TWO

- Supine.
- The therapist sits facing the side of the patient. The occiput rests in the therapist's superior hand. Thumb and index finger of caudal hand gently grip the lateral aspects of the hyoid bone.

TREATMENT: PHASE TWO

1. *First Plane:* Move occiput and hyoid bone in opposite directions: medial/lateral. Move in the direction of ease.
2. *Second Plane:* Now add or "stack" the second plane movements. Move occiput and hyoid bone in opposite directions: anterior/posterior. Move in the direction of ease.
3. *Third Plane:* Now add or "stack" the third plane. Move occiput and hyoid bone in opposite directions: right/left rotation (clockwise/counterclockwise). Move in the direction of ease.
4. *The Release:* Maintain the fulcrum created in Steps 1 to 4. As the tissue unwinds and movement occurs in the body's internal environment, there is a temptation to move the hands and release the fulcrum. *Resist the temptation to release the fulcrum.*

POSITION: PHASE THREE

- Supine.
- The therapist sits facing the side of the patient. The occiput rests in the therapist's superior hand. The humb and index finger of the caudal hand gently grip the lateral borders of the thyroid cartilage.

TREATMENT: PHASE THREE

1. *First Plane:* Move the occiput and thyroid cartilage in opposite directions: medial/lateral.

2. *Second Plane:* Move occiput and thyroid cartilage in opposite directions: right/left rotation.

3. *Third Plane:* Move occiput and thyroid cartilage in opposite directions: right/left sidebending.

4. Go indirect: 3-planar indirect direction of ease. Maintain the fulcrum.

POSITION: PHASE FOUR

- Supine.
- The therapist sits facing the side of the patient. Grip gently in one hand the lateral aspects of the hyoid bone. Grip the lateral borders of the thyroid cartilage in the other hand.

TREATMENT: PHASE FOUR

1. *First Plane:* Move occiput and thyroid cartilage in opposite directions: medial/lateral. Move in the direction of ease.

2. *Second Plane:* Now add or "stack" the second plane movements. Move occiput and thyroid cartilage in opposite directions: anterior/posterior. Move in the direction of ease.

3. *Third Plane:* Now add or "stack" the third plane. Move occiput and thyroid cartilage in opposite directions: right/left rotation (clockwise/counterclockwise). Move in the direction of ease.

4. *The Release:* Maintain the fulcrum created in Steps 1 to 4. As the tissue unwinds and movement occurs in the body's internal environment, there is a temptation to move the hands and release the fulcrum. *Resist the temptation to release the fulcrum.*

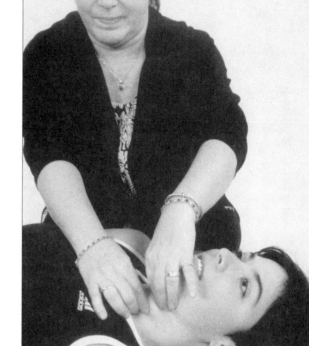

Figure 72. Hand position for Phase 4 of the Hyoid Release.

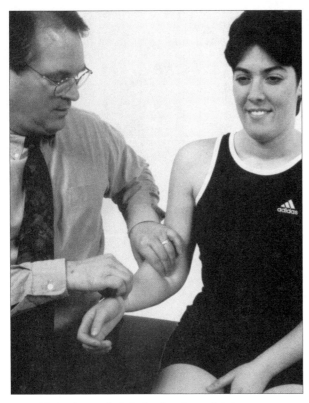

Figure 73. Hand position for Radioulnar Joint Hanging Technique.

Fascial Release for the Radioulnar Joint: A Hanging Technique

INDICATION

Limitation of motion in supination and pronation; anterior compartment syndrome; carpal tunnel syndrome.

APPLICATION

The technique is performed after an application of a general Soft Tissue Myofascial Release.

POSITION

- Sitting.
- The patient's elbow is flexed to 90 degrees. The therapist firmly grips the *radius bone* at both ends, distal to the elbow and proximal to the wrist.

TREATMENT

1. Grip as firmly as necessary to hold the fulcrum without inching.
2. Hold onto the radius; the rest of the forearm "hangs" from the radius.
3. *The Release:* The interosseous membrane will unwind.

Fascial Release for the Tibiofibular Joint: A Hanging Technique

INDICATION

Limitation of motion in tibial rotation, knee flexion and extension, and ankle dorsiflexion.

APPLICATION

The technique is performed after an application of a general Soft Tissue Myofascial Release.

POSITION

- Supine.
- The hip is flexed to 45 degrees. The knee is flexed to 90 degrees. The therapist sits at the side of the table. The therapist's hands loosely hold the distal leg while the therapist's elbows rest on the table. The therapist's caudal hand holds the heel loosely to keep the leg from rotation while the distal fibula rests on the thumb of the caudal hand. The superior hand holds the calf while the superior fibula (just caudal to the fibular head) rests on the thumb.

TREATMENT

1. Grip as firmly as necessary to hold the fulcrum without inching.
2. Hold on to the fibula while the tibia "hangs."
3. *The Release*: The interosseous membrane will unwind.

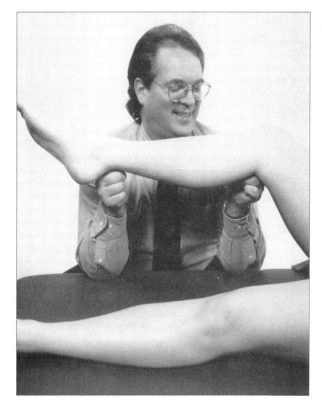

Figure 74. Hand position for Tibiofibular Hanging Technique.

Cervico-Thoracic Junction: A Specific Soft Tissue Fascial Release Technique

POSITION

- Supine.
- The therapist sits at the head of the patient.
- One hand is under the cervico-thoracic junction; the spinous processes of C7/T1 lie in the palm of that hand. The other hand lies on top of the patient: palm faced down. The thenar and hypothenar eminences contact supraclavicular tissue. The thumb and fingers are spread out so that there is contact on all structures and tissues: supraclavicular tissue; sternum; clavicles; bilateral ribs.

TREATMENT

1. The hands compress together gently (not enough pressure to burst a soap bubble).

2. *First Plane:* One hand moves the tissues/structures cephalad; the other hand moves the tissues/structures caudad. Move in the direction of ease.

3. *Second Plane:* Now add or "stack" the second plane movements. One hand moves the tissues/structures to the right; the other distorts the tissues/structures to the left. Move in the direction of ease.

4. *Third Plane:* Now add or "stack" the third plane. One hand moves the tissues clockwise; the other hand works them counterclockwise.

5. *The Release:* Maintain the fulcrum created in Steps 1 to 4. As the tissue unwinds and movement occurs in the body's internal environment, there is a temptation to move the hands and release the fulcrum. *Resist the temptation to release the fulcrum.*

CHAPTER 19

SPECIALIZED MYOFASCIAL RELEASE TECHNIQUE FOR FACIAL EXPRESSION

Ocular Expression Release

POSITION

- Place fingers around both eyeballs. (See Figures 74 and 75.)

TREATMENT

1. Turn the eyeballs clockwise, then counterclockwise, with no more than a force of 1 gram.

2. Determine the direction(s) of greater mobility. Either eyeball may be more mobile in the same or opposite direction than the other.

3. Turn the eyeballs in the direction(s) of greater mobility up to the barrier. Return to inter-barrier zone, before the barrier (maintaining no more than 1 gram of force).

4. Push eyeballs posterior, into orbits, to the inter-barrier zone with no more than 1 gram of force.

5. Maintain the fulcrum for fascial unwinding.

Note: All clockwise and counterclockwise rotations of the tissue must be pure circular movements. No sagittal or transverse plane movements are indicated, only pure coronal plane movements. All facial expression is clockwise/counterclockwise motion.

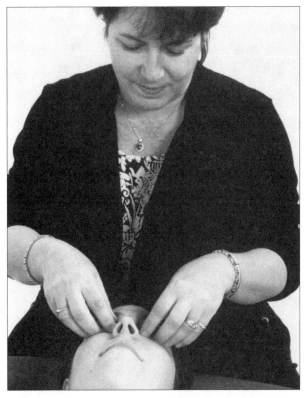

Figure 75. Therapist and patient position for the Ocular Expression Release.

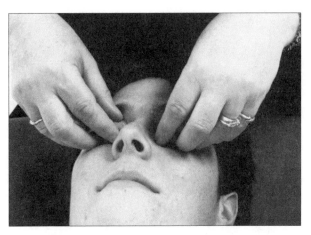

Figure 76. Hand placements for the Ocular Expression Release.

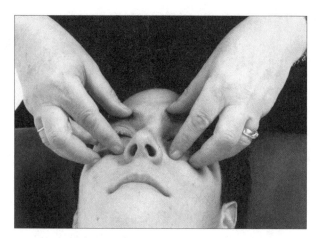

Figure 77. Hand placements for the Orbit Expression Release.

Orbit Expression Release

POSITION

- Place finger tips on the orbit; surround the eyeballs.

TREATMENT

1. Assess and treat both orbits together.
2. Spread the orbits: fingertips push on cranial and facial bones to "open" orbits wider in all dimensions. Use a force of no more than 5 grams.
3. Rotate orbits clockwise and counterclockwise. (Maintain a force of no more than 5 grams.)
4. Determine the direction(s) of greater mobility. (Either of the two orbits may be more mobile in the same or opposite directions.)
5. Rotate the orbits in the directions of greater mobility up to the inter-barrier zone. The fingers are still pushing on the orbits, maintaining the spread of the orbits attained in Step 2. (Maintain a force of no more than 5 grams.)
6. Maintain the fulcrum for fascial unwinding.

Note: All clockwise and counterclockwise rotations of the tissues must be pure circular movement. No sagittal or transverse plane movements are indicated, only pure coronal plane movement. All facial expression is clockwise/counterclockwise motion.

Lips Expression Release

POSITION

- Place the fingers of one hand on the top lip; place the fingers of the other hand on the bottom lip.

TREATMENT

1. Rotate each lip clockwise and counterclockwise up to the inter-barrier zone with a force of no more than 5 grams.

2. Determine the direction(s) of greater mobility. (Either of the two lips may be more mobile in the same or opposite directions.)

3. Rotate the lips in the direction of greater mobility up to the inter-barrier zone. Maintain a force of no more than 5 grams.

4. Spread the lips to make them "longer." (Maintain a force of no more than 5 grams.)

5. Maintain fulcrum for fascial unwinding.

Note: All clockwise and counterclockwise rotation of the tissue must be pure circular movements. No sagittal or transverse plane movements are indicated, only pure coronal plane movements. All facial expression is clockwise/counterclockwise motion.

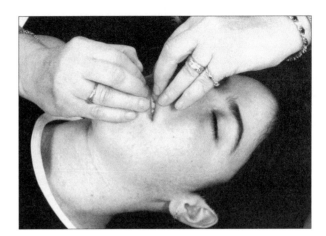

Figure 78. Hand placements for the Lips Expression Release.

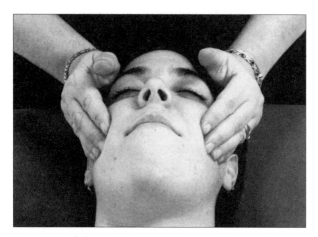

Figure 79. Hand placements for the Cheeks Expression Release.

Cheeks Expression Release

POSITION

- Place the fingers of both hands just inferior to the *zygoma*.

TREATMENT

1. Press the soft tissue gently, posterior/medial with a force of no more than 5 grams.
2. Lengthen the tissue by stretching superior/inferior. The fingers are inferior to the zygoma, the thumbs are on the superior aspect of the inferior border of the mandible. Fingers and thumbs stretch the tissue by spreading apart from each other. Maintain a force of no more than 5 grams.
3. Maintain the stretch (superior/inferior) of the soft tissue. Rotate the tissue clockwise and counterclockwise. Maintain a force of no more than 5 grams.
4. Determine the direction(s) of greater mobility. (The tissue of either side may have greater mobility in the same or opposite directions.)
5. Rotate the tissue in the direction of greater mobility up to the inter-barrier zone. Maintain a force of no more than 5 grams.
6. Maintain fulcrum for fascial unwinding.

Note: All clockwise and counterclockwise rotation of the tissue must be pure circular movements. No sagittal or transverse plane movements are indicated, only pure coronal plane movements. All facial expression is clockwise/counterclockwise motion.

Forehead Expression Release

POSITION

- Place the fingers along the length of the eyebrows.

TREATMENT

1. Rotate the eyebrows clockwise and counterclockwise with a force of no more than 5 grams.

2. Determine the direction(s) of greater mobility. (Either side may have greater mobility in the same or opposite direction(s).)

3. Rotate the tissue in the direction of greater mobility up to the inter-barrier zone. (Maintain a force of no more than 5 grams).

4. Maintain the fulcrum for fascial unwinding.

Note: All clockwise and counterclockwise rotation of the tissue must be pure circular movements. No sagittal or transverse plane movements are indicated, only pure coronal plane movements. All facial expression is clockwise/counterclockwise motion.

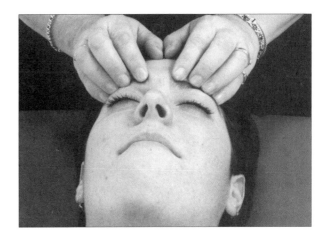

Figure 80. Hand placements for the Forehead Expression Release.

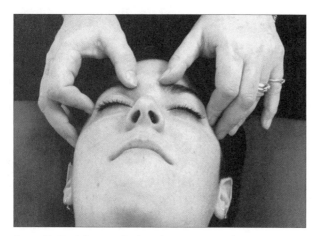

Figure 81. Hand placements for the Eyebrows Expression Release.

Eyebrows Expression Release

POSITION

- Place the thumbs and index fingers on both ends of eyebrows.

TREATMENT

1. Stretch the eyebrows up to the inter-barrier zone with a force of no more than 5 grams.
2. Push the eyebrows forcefully inferior and towards the orbits but without contact on the eyeballs.
3. Push the eyebrows into the inferior aspect of the superior orbit. CAUTION: place *no* pressure on the eyeball.
4. Rotate the tissue clockwise and counterclockwise. Maintain a force of no more than 5 grams.
5. Determine the direction(s) of greater mobility. (Either side may have greater mobility in the same or opposite direction(s).)
6. Rotate the tissue in the direction of greater mobility up to the inter-barrier zone. Maintain a force of no more than 5 grams.
8. Maintain fulcrum for fascial unwinding.

Note: All clockwise and counterclockwise rotation of the tissue must be pure circular movements. No sagittal or transverse plane movements are indicated, only pure coronal plane movements. All facial expression is clockwise/counterclockwise motion.

Tongue Expression Release

POSITION

- Grasp both ends of the hyoid bone with the thumb and index finger of one hand.
- The thumb and index finger of the other hand grasps both angles of the mandible.

TREATMENT

1. Rotate the hyoid bone clockwise and counterclockwise with a force of no more than 5 grams.

2. Determine the direction of greater mobility of the hyoid bone.

3. Rotate the hyoid bone in the direction of greater mobility up to the inter-barrier zone. Maintain no more than 5 grams of force.

4. Squeeze the angles of the mandible medial. Maintain no more than 5 grams of force.

5. Maintain fulcrum for fascial unwinding.

Note: All clockwise and counterclockwise rotation of the tissue must be pure circular movements. No sagittal or transverse plane movements are indicated, only pure coronal plane movements. All facial expression is clockwise/counterclockwise motion.

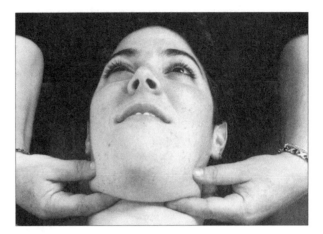

Figure 82. Alternate hand placement for the Tongue Expression Release.

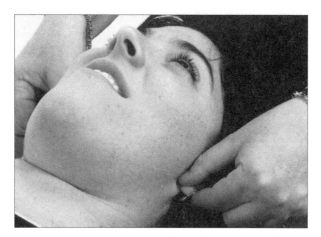

Figure 83. Hand placement for the Ears Expression Release.

Ears Expression Release

POSITION

- Place the index finger and thumb of each hand at the lobes of the ears.

TREATMENT

1. Squeeze the ear lobes medial/lateral (*not* anterior/posterior) with a force of no more than 5 grams.

2. Turn the earlobes inward. When the earlobe is squeezed, the finger can be over the *meatus* (opening) of the ear.

3. Rotate the tissue surrounding the meatus clockwise and counterclockwise. Maintain no more than 5 grams of force.

4. Determine the direction(s) of greater mobility. (The directions of greater mobility for each ear may be the same or different relative to the other.)

5. Rotate the tissue in the direction of greater mobility. Maintain no more than 5 grams of force.

6. Maintain fulcrum for fascial unwinding.

Note: All clockwise and counterclockwise rotation of the tissue must be pure circular movements. No sagittal or transverse plane movements are indicated, only pure coronal plane movements. All facial expression is clockwise/counterclockwise motion.

Smile Expression Release

POSITION

- Place the index finger and thumb of one hand just slightly inside the mouth at the lateral edges of the inner lips. Use finger cots or glove.

TREATMENT

1. Stretch the lateral edges of the mouth up to the inter-barrier zone with a force of no more than 5 grams.

2. Maintain the stretch of the tissue. Rotate the tissue clockwise and counterclockwise. Maintain no more than 5 grams of force.

3. Determine the direction of greater mobility. Index finger and thumb will rotate together in the same direction.

4. Rotate the tissue in the direction of greater mobility up to the inter-barrier zone. Maintain no more than 5 grams of force.

5. Maintain fulcrum for fascial unwinding.

Note: All clockwise and counterclockwise rotation of the tissue must be pure circular movements. No sagittal or transverse plane movements are indicated, only pure coronal plane movements. All facial expression is clockwise/counterclockwise motion.

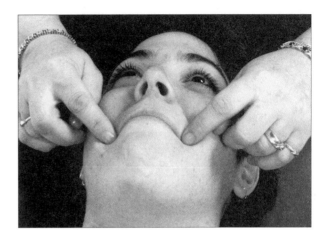

Figure 84. Hand placements for the Smile Expression Release.

Crying Expression Release

POSITION

- Place thumbs at the lateral edges of both orbits.
- Place both index fingers just slightly inside the mouth at the lateral edges of the lips. Use finger cots or gloves.

TREATMENT

1. Stretch the index fingers and thumbs apart: superior/inferior stretch up to the inter-barrier zone with a force of no more than 5 grams.
2. Maintain the stretch. Rotate the thumb and index finger of each hand in clockwise and counterclockwise rotations. Maintain no more than 5 grams of force.
3. Determine the direction(s) of greater mobility. (Either the right or left side tissue may have greater mobility in the same or opposite direction.)
4. Rotate the tissue in the direction of greater mobility up to the inter-barrier zone. Maintain no more than 5 grams of force.
5. Maintain the fulcrum for fascial unwinding.

Note: All clockwise and counterclockwise rotation of the tissue must be pure circular movements. No sagittal or transverse plane movements are indicated, only pure coronal plane movements. All facial expression is clockwise/counterclockwise motion.

Lustre Expression Release

POSITION

- Place hands (palms) on the right and left sides of the face.

TREATMENT

1. Rotate the tissues clockwise and counterclockwise with a force of no more than 5 grams.
2. Determine the directions of greater mobility. (Either the right or left side may have greater mobility in the same or opposite directions.)
3. Rotate the tissue in the direction of greater mobility up to the inter-barrier zone. Maintain no more than 5 grams of force.
4. Maintain the fulcrum for fascial unwinding.

Note: All clockwise and counterclockwise rotation of the tissue must be pure circular movements. No sagittal or transverse plane movements are indicated, only pure coronal plane movements. All facial expression is clockwise/counterclockwise motion.

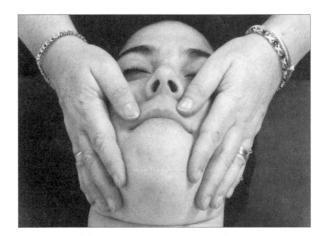

Figure 85. Hand placements for the Lustre Expression Release.

CHAPTER 20

THE RESPIRATORY DIAPHRAGM SYSTEM
MYOFASCIAL RELEASE OF TRANSVERSE FASCIAL RESTRICTIONS

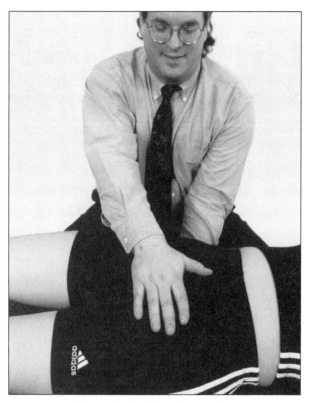

Figure 86. Hand placements for the Pelvic Diaphragm Release.

The transverse fascial releases are essential for all patients. These techniques can be repeated every several treatment sessions.

Pelvic Diaphragm Release

POSITION

- Supine.
- The therapist sits at the side, facing the patient.
- The sacrum is in the palm of the bottom hand. The top hand faces palm down with a finger on the pubic bone and the rest of the fingers on the suprapubic and lower abdominal soft tissues.

TREATMENT

1. Compress the *pelvic diaphragm region* with both hands, squeezing gently, imaging a soap bubble between the hands. Don't burst the bubble. Maintain gentle compression.

2. *First Plane:* The anterior hand moves cephalad while the posterior hand moves caudal, distorting the soap bubble. The hands return to neutral and reverse directions: the anterior hand moves the tissue caudal, while the posterior hand move the tissue cephalad. Consider which directions (cephalad/caudal of caudal/cephalad) have the greatest mobility and least resistance. Let the hands move the tissue in the indirect direction of ease. Keep the hands in that new position. Maintain those directions of forces on the tissues.

3. *Second Plane:* Now add or "stack" the second plane movements. Do not return the

hands on tissues to neutral. Move the tissues under the anterior hand medially while the posterior hand moves the tissues laterally. Return the tissues to neutral and compare the ease of tissue mobility when the anterior hand moves the tissue laterally while the posterior hand moves the tissues medially.

4. *Third Plane:* Now add or "stack" the third plane. Do not return the tissues to neutral; they are displaced form neutral on two planes now. Move the tissues with the anterior hand in a clockwise direction, while the posterior hand moves the tissues in a counterclockwise direction. Then return the tissues to neutral on this plane. Compare the opposite tissue distortion pattern. Move the tissues counterclockwise with the anterior hand while the posterior hand moves the tissues clockwise. Compare the two different tissue distortion patterns: clockwise/counterclockwise or counterclockwise/clockwise. Which indirect pattern has the greatest mobility? Return the tissues to that direction of distortion. Now there are three directions of forces from each hand onto the tissues; each hand is displacing the tissues on three planes.

5. *The Fulcrum:* There are now four directions of forces from each hand onto the body.

   - Slight compression
   - Coronal plane: clockwise or counter-clockwise
   - Transverse plane: medial or lateral
   - Sagittal plane: superior or inferior

The intersection of these eight forces is a "fixed point." This fixed point is the *fulcrum* around which the fascial tissue will *unwind*. This fulcrum is the mechanoenergetic interface for the 3-Planar Myofascial Fulcrum Technique.

6. *The Release:* Maintain the fulcrum. The hands do not move. They do not follow the tissue movements, although the temptation to move the hands and follow the tissue motion will be great. The goal is not a physiologic unwinding of a body part. The objective is the internal "unraveling" of the fascial tissue. By maintaining the fulcrum, energy will be created/transduced. The force of the energy causing the fascial release will produce more changes in the internal environment of the connective tissue. The fascial unwinding will be slow and gentle. Do not allow quick or repetitive or forceful physiologic movements.

If the patient begins to move any body part quickly, without repetition, or with force, say to the patient: "Please don't move in that manner." If the body part changes position in space slowly and gently in order to facilitate the internal tissue unwinding, this movement is acceptable. At the end of the release, the hands will be in different positions because of the unwinding of the internal body tissues. The body parts that experienced the internal tissue unwinding will be in a more normal anatomical, neutral position.

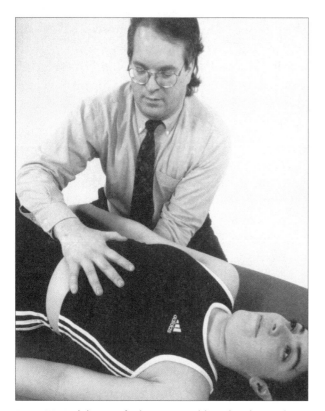

Figure 87. Hand placements for the Respiratory Abdominal Diaphragm Release.

Respiratory Abdominal Diaphragm Release

POSITION

- Supine.
- The therapist sits on one side, facing the patient.
- The spinous processes of T12/L1 lie in the palm of the bottom hand. The top hand lies palm down, over the lower rib cage. Some of the top hand and fingers contact the sternum, the bilateral ribs, and infracostal soft tissue.

TREATMENT

1. Compress the *abdominal respiratory diaphragm* with both hands, squeezing gently, imaging a soap bubble between the hands. Don't burst the bubble. Maintain the gentle compression.

2. *First Plane:* The anterior hand moves cephalad while the posterior hand moves caudal, distoring the soap bubble. The hands return to neutral and reverse direction: the anterior hand moves the tissue caudal, while the posterior hand moves the tissue cephalad. Consider which direction (cephalad/caudal or caudal/cephalad) has the greatest mobility and the least resistance. The hands move the tissues in the "indirect" direction of ease. Keep hands in that new position, maintaining those directions of forces on the tissues.

3. *Second Plane:* Now add or "stack" the second plane. Do not return the hands on the tissues to neutral. Move the tissues under the anterior hand medially while the posterior hand moves the tissues laterally. Return the tissues to neutral and compare the ease of tissue mobility when the anterior hand moves the tissue laterally while the posterior hand moves the tissue medially.

Consider which directions (medial/lateral or lateral/medial) are the most mobile, least restricted. Return the tissues to that position. Maintain these directions of forces on the tissues, as well as those forces from the first plane.

4. *Third Plane:* Now add or "stack" the third plane. Do not return the tissues to neutral; they are displaced from neutral on two planes now. Move the tissues with the anterior hand in a clockwise direction while the posterior hand moves the tissues in a counterclockwise direction. Then return the tissues to neutral on this plane. Compare the opposite tissue distortion pattern. Move the tissue counterclockwise with the anterior hand while the posterior hand moves the tissue clockwise. Compare the two different tissue distortion patterns (clockwise/counterclockwise or counterclockwise/clockwise). Which is the indirect pattern with the greatest mobility? Return the tissue to that direction of distortion. Now there are three planes of forces from each hand onto the tissues. Each hand is displacing the tissues on three planes.

5. *The Fulcrum:* There are now four directions of forces from each hand onto the body.

   - Slight compression
   - Coronal plane: clockwise or counter-clockwise
   - Transverse plane: medial or lateral
   - Sagittal plane: superior or inferior

The intersection of these eight forces is a "fixed point." This fixed point is the *fulcrum* around which the fascial tissue will *unwind*. This fulcrum is the mechanoenergetic interface for the 3-Planar Myofascial Fulcrum Technique.

6. *The Release:* Maintain the fulcrum. The hands do not move. They do not follow the tissue movements, although the temptation to move the hands and follow the tissue motion will be great. The goal is not a physiologic unwinding of a body part. The objective is the internal "unraveling" of the fascial tissue. By maintaining the fulcrum, energy will be created/transduced. The force of the energy causing the fascial release will produce more changes in the internal environment of the connective tissue. The fascial unwinding will be slow and gentle. Do not allow quick or repetitive or forceful physiologic movements.

If the patient begins to move any body part quickly, without repetition, or with force, say to the patient: "Please don't move in that manner." If the body part changes position in space slowly and gently in order to facilitate the internal tissue unwinding, this movement is acceptable. At the end of the release, the hands will be in different positions because of the unwinding of the internal body tissues. The body parts that experienced the internal tissue unwinding will be in a more normal anatomical, neutral position.

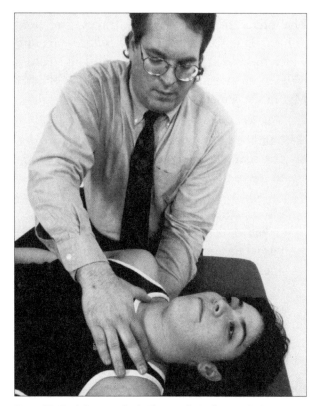

Figure 88. Hand placements for the Thoracic Inlet Diaphragm Release.

Thoracic Inlet Diaphragm Release

POSITION

- Supine.
- Therapist sits at the side, facing patient.
- The spinous processes of C7/T1 lie in the palm of the bottom hand. The top hand lies palm down over the thoracic inlet. Hand and some fingers make contact with supra-clavicular soft tissue, clavicles, sternum, and bilateral ribs.

TREATMENT

1. Compress the *thoracic inlet diaphragm* with both hands, squeezing gently, imaging a soap bubble between the hands. Don't burst the bubble! Maintain the gentle compression.

2. *First Plane:* The anterior hand moves cephalad while the posterior hand moves caudal, distorting the soap bubble. The hands return to neutral and reverse directions. The anterior hand moves the tissue caudal, while the posterior hand moves the tissue cephalad. Consider which directions (cephalad/caudal or caudal/cephalad) has the greatest mobility and least resistance. The hands move the tissue in the "indirect" direction of ease. Keep hands in that new position, maintaining those directions of forces on the tissues.

3. *Second Plane:* Now add or "stack" the second plane movements. Do not return the hands or tissues to neutral. Move the tissues under the anterior hand medially, while the posterior hand moves the tissue laterally. Return the tissues to neutral and compare the ease of tissue mobility when the anterior hand moves the tissues laterally while the posterior hand moves the tissue medially. Consider which directions (medial/lateral or

lateral/medial) were the most mobile, the least restricted. Return the tissue to that position. Maintain these directions of forces on the tissues as well as those forces from the first plane.

4. *Third Plane:* Now add or "stack" the third plane. Do not return the tissues to neutral; they are displaced from neutral on two planes now. Move the tissue with the anterior hand in a clockwise direction, while the posterior hand moves the tissues in a counterclockwise direction. Then return the tissues to neutral on this plane. Compare the opposite tissue distortion pattern. Move the tissues counterclockwise with the anterior hand while the posterior hand moves the tissues clockwise. Compare the two different tissue-distorting patterns (clockwise/counterclockwise or counterclockwise/clockwise). Which was the indirect pattern-the one with the greatest mobility? Return the tissue to that direction of distortion. Now there are three directions of forces from each hand onto the tissues; each hand is displacing the tissues on three planes.

5. *The Fulcrum:* There are now four directions of forces from each hand onto the body.

   - Slight compression
   - Coronal plane: clockwise or counter-clockwise
   - Transverse plane: medial or lateral
   - Sagittal plane: superior or inferior

The intersection of these eight forces is a "fixed point." This fixed point is the *fulcrum* around which the fascial tissue will *unwind*. This fulcrum is the mechanoenergetic interface for the 3-Planar Myofascial Fulcrum Technique.

5. *The Release:* Maintain the fulcrum. The hands do not move. They do not follow the tissue movements, although the temptation to move the hands and follow the tissue motion will be great. The goal is not a physiologic unwinding of a body part. The objective is the internal "unraveling" of the fascial tissue. By maintaining the fulcrum, energy will be created/transduced. The force of the energy causing the fascial release will produce more changes in the internal environment of the connective tissue. The fascial unwinding will be slow and gentle. Do not allow quick or repetitive or forceful physiologic movements.

If the patient begins to move any body part quickly, without repetition, or with force, say to the patient: "Please don't move in that manner." If the body part changes position in space slowly and gently in order to facilitate the internal tissue unwinding, this movement is acceptable. At the end of the release, the hands will be in different positions because of the unwinding of the internal body tissues. The body parts that experienced the internal tissue unwinding will be in a more normal anatomical, neutral position.

CHAPTER 21

GENERAL PROTOCOL FOR MYOFASCIAL RELEASE

EVALUATION

1. Static Posture
2. Dynamic Posture
3. Myofascial Glide
4. Myofascial Mapping

APPLICATION

1. Myofascial Release is most effective and efficient when performed after biomechanical dysfunction of the pelvic joints, sacrum, spine and the occipito-atlantal joint have been treated once with Muscle Energy and Beyond Techniques.

2. Myofascial Release is most effective and efficient, and least aggressive to the patient, when performed after severe protective muscle spasm has been eliminated with Jones' Strain and Counterstrain Technique.

3. These Myofascial Release techniques can be utilized on all severe chronic neurologic patients such as coma patients and patients in persistent vegetative state. Even with severe contractures, the therapist can initiate a program of structural rehabilitation.

TREATMENT

1. General Soft Tissue Myofascial Release to body areas indicated by evaluation
2. Progression:
    ▪ Proximal before distal
    ▪ Most severe asymmetry before least asymmetry
    ▪ Static before dynamic

   ▪ "Take up the slack" of superficial tissues and treat deeper tissues
   ▪ Soft Tissue Myofascial Release before Articular Myofascial Release

3. Articular Myofascial Release for the pelvic joints: anterior and posterior releases
4. Articular Myofascial Release for the sacrum
5. Soft Tissue and Articular Myofascial Release for the thoracolumbar junction
6. Myofascial Release for the cervicothoracic junction
7. Defacilitation of the spine
8. Lumbosacral decompression
9. Release of extradural impingement from lumbosacral decompression
10. Cranio-cervical release
11. Release of extradural impingements from cranio-cervical release
12. Balance of cranial dura: lateral vault hold and fronto-occipital hold
13. Myofascial Release for the hyoid system
14. Peripheral Joint: Articular Myofascial Release as needed (proximal to distal)
15. Special Techniques: Muscle belly, scars, ligaments, tendons, capsules

Consider using the form on the following page to either track progress of a treatment plan, or to document treatment recommendations.

Note number of sessions (either completed or recommended). Use diagram to note body parts.

Myofascial Release Treatment

Patient _____ Date _____

☐ Soft Tissue Myofascial Release Technique (Fulcrum Technique)

☐ Articular Fascial Release Technique for the iliosacral joints: anterior and posterior

☐ Articular Fascial Release Technique for the sacrum
  _____ *sessions*

☐ Articular Fascial Release Technique for L5/S1
  _____ *sessions*

☐ Soft Tissue and Articular Myofascial Release for the thoracolumbar junction
  _____ *sessions*

☐ Myofascial Release for the cervico-thoracic junction
  _____ *sessions*

☐ Defacilitation of the spine
  comment: _____
  _____

☐ Lumbosacral decompression
  comment: _____
  _____

☐ Release of extradural impingements from lumbosacral decompression
  _____ *sessions*

☐ Cranio-cervical release
  _____ *sessions*

☐ Temporomandibular joint compression and decompression
  _____ *sessions*

☐ Release of extradural impingements from cranio-cervical release
  _____ *sessions*

☐ Balance of the cranial dura: lateral volt hold and fronto-occipital hold
  _____ *sessions*

☐ Myofascial Release for the hyoid system (4 phases).
  comment: _____
  _____

☐ Peripheral joints: Articular Fascial Release

☐ Transverse Fascial Release (all diaphragms):
  _____ *sessions*
  comment: _____
  _____

PART FOUR

ASSESSMENT WITH POSTURAL ANALYSIS, FASCIAL GLIDE, AND MYOFASCIAL MAPPING

CHAPTER 22

EVALUATION OF POSTURE
INDICATIONS FOR TREATMENT WITH MYOFASCIAL RELEASE

Postural deviations are reflections of joint and soft tissue dysfunction. Posture is evaluated on a sagittal plane, coronal plane, and transverse plane. It is important to stand with a neutral base of support during all posture evaluations. The feet should be acetabular distance apart with approximately 15 to 20 degrees of equal rotation for the feet. (See Figures 89 and 80.) It is important to note that one foot is not slightly in front of the other. The knees should be equally flexed/ extended. If there is recurvatum of one knee, it should be maintained in neutral to equal the posture of the other knee

Sagittal Plane Posture

Sagittal plane posture is assessed from a side view. (See Figure 91.) Sagittal plane movements are flexion and extension. If the patient can stand with fair standing balance, the practitioner can image an imaginary plumbline, which touches the apex of a normal *kyphosis*. This plumbline should also touch the occiput and the buttocks. The distance from this plumbline to the apex of the *lumbar lordosis* is approximately five centimeters in healthy sagittal plane posture. The distance of this plumbline to the apex of the *cervical lordosis* should be approximately 6 cm.

Typical postural dysfunction includes a flexed lumbar spine and a forward head and neck, which is a flexed cervical spine. Occasionally, the therapist views an apparent excessive lumbar lordosis, which is often an indication of dysfunction of the lumbosacral junction and the sacroiliac joint rather than excessive lumbar extension. A posture which appears to be an excessive cervical lordosis is typically the result of a hyperextended occipito/atlantal joint, which is compensatory for the hyperflexed cervical spine. If the distance from

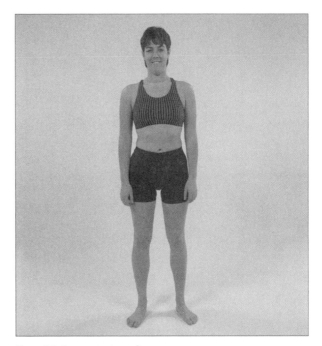

Figure 89. Anterior view in standing.

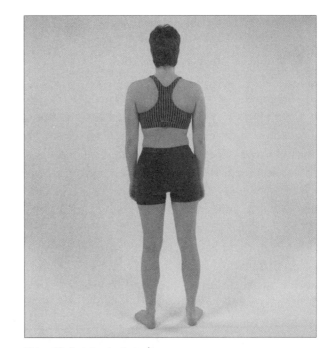

Figure 90. Posterior view in standing.

133

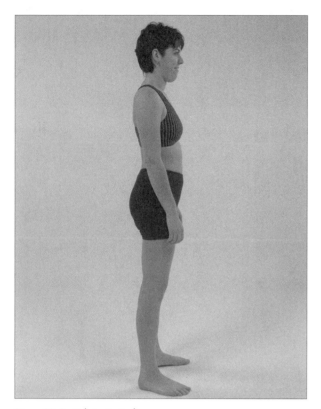

Figure 91. Sagittal view in standing.

the apex of the cervical lordosis to the imaginary plumbline exceeds 6 cm, this reflects an increase in the flexion of the cervical intervertebral joints. Anterior shears of the cervical vertebral bodies, especially C7 on T1, often accompany forward head and neck posture. (Caillet describes this dysfunction).

When the cervical spine is flexed, there is a natural tendency for the eyes to look to the floor. The need for an extension of the occiput on the atlas in order to see straight ahead is greater when there greater the flexion of the cervical spine. This hyperextension of the occiput on the atlas compromises the suboccipital space, which should be 9 to 12 mm. As the suboccipital space is compromised, there is compression of the neurovascular bundle, including cranial nerves: 9, 10, 11, and 12. Circulation to the head can be affected. With a forward head and neck posture, together with hyperextension of the occipito-atlantal joint, there is stretching and lengthening of the anterior

cervical and hyoid musculature. Kinesiologically, this affects the strength and function of the anterior cervical and tongue musculature. The flexibility of the connective tissue, which surrounds the larynx and pharnyx, is affected, and fascial dysfunction at the anterior neck results. Swallowing can be affected. The stretch of the anterior cervical soft tissue will pull on the mandible. In order to maintain a resting closed mouth, the masticatory muscles are maintained in a state of contraction, eliciting protective muscle spasm. Typically, with a forward head and neck posture, these in lengthening and weakening of the anterior cervical soft tissue and hyoid muscles, hypertonicity of the masticatory muscles and hypertonicity of the suboccipital musculature which maintains occiput in an extend position.

In the sagittal plane postural evaluation, there may be an excessive kyphosis, or a regional loss of thoracic kyphosis. At the pelvis and hips, there may be excessive flexion of the hip joints. The posture of the peripheral joints on a saggital plane can also be assessed. Knee recurvatum is a common postural dysfunction of the lower extremities. Posterior displacement of the distal tibial articular surface on talus is also common.

The static postural evaluation can be interpreted, and will indicate limitations in physiologic ranges of motion. Fryette documented three laws of biomechanics. Application of his third law explains how static postural dysfunction affects dynamic movement. Fryette noted that when movement is taken up on any one plane, the potential for movement in all other planes is reduced. With neuromusculoskeletal dysfunction, which results in limitations in range of motion and joint hypomobility, there is postural dysfunction. This means that there is a region of the body which is not maintained in a resting anatomic neutral position, but rests, at least in one plane. For example, consider the neck held in right sidebending. Fryette's third law implies that if the neck is stuck in right sidebending (on a coronal plane), the potential for a full range of motion on a sagittal or a transverse plane is compromised. Also, if the static postural evaluation presents with a forward head and neck posture due to cervical flexed vertebrae, there can possibly be full cervical flexion; there cannot be full cervical extension.

Evaluating physiologic movement of cervical spine extension is especially difficult, yet important. Normal occipito-atlantal joint extension is 15 degrees. This joint has 15 degrees of flexion and 15 degrees of extension. (Chin tuck will give 15 degrees of occipitoatlantal joint flexion; chin protrusion will give 15 degrees of occipitoatlantal joint extension). *A common clinical assessment error is allowing excessive protrusion of the chin during flexion and extension.* A maximum of 15 degrees extension of the occipitoatlantal joint should be maintained, and cervical extension one segment at a time down the kinetic chain should be assessed. *The common compensatory (trick) movement at the cervical spine is anterior shearing of the vertebral bodies. This means, when there is limitation of cervical extension, the cervical segments will compensate by shearing anteriorly in order to attain an extended head and neck posture.* The most significant anterior shearing typically occurs at C7 on T1, the cervicothoracic junction. If anterior shears of any or all of the cervical segments are present, cervical movement will be limited in all physiologic ranges of motion, because this is a pathologic position for the vertebral bodies.

Per definition, during extension, the body part extending must be totally posterior to midline. Per definition, during flexion, the body part flexing must be completely anterior to midline. This means, if during cervical extension, any part of the anterior neck is more anterior to midline than when in neutral resting position, the movement is not true extension.

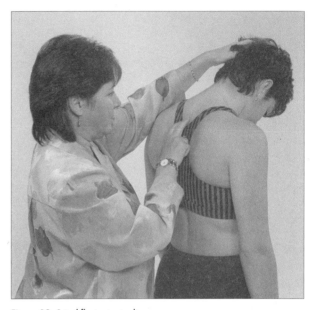

Figure 92. Spinal flexion in standing.

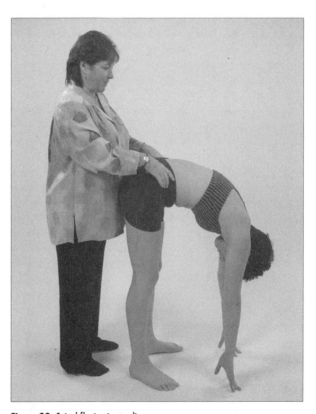

Figure 93. Spinal flexion in standing.

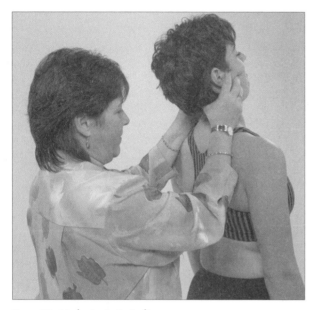

Figure 94. Spinal extension in standing.

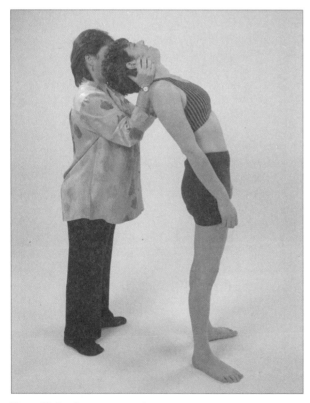

Figure 95. Spinal extension in standing.

Lumbar flexion and extension can also be assessed. (See Figures 93 and 95.) With typical postural dysfunction of lumbar hyperflexion (decreased lumbar lordosis), lumbar extension will be limited in range of motion. When there is lumbosacral junction dysfunction and sacroiliac joint dysfunction, lumbar flexion and extension will be limited.

Physiologic movement of the cervical, thoracic, and lumbar spine can be assed through full ranges of motion in flexions and extension. Severe dysfunction will be noted in inner ranges of motion. Moderate dysfunction will be notes in mid range of motion. Mild dysfunction will be noted in outer ranges of motion. Often the trunk will deviate from midline during flexion and extension to compensate for neuromusculoskeletal dysfunction that is affecting sagittal plane movement. Sagittal plane postural dysfunction is best evaluated in standing, but it is important to assess segmental vertebral movement. Typical compensatory (trick) movements during lumbar flexion include excessive posterior tibial glide on talus (plantar flexion) with excessive hip flexion. A typical compensatory movement during lumbar extension is hip extension. Sitting is an alternative assessment position. Supine and prone are more difficult positions for evaluation of postural dysfunction on a sagittal plane.

Coronal Plane Posture

Coronal plane posture can be evaluated in the standing position (See Figures 96 and 97.). Either a posterior view or an anterior view is appropriate and will typically provide the same information. If the patient cannot stand, then coronal plane posture in sitting, supine, and prone position is still possible.

The patient is standing with feet acetabular distance apart, with approximately 15 to 20 degrees of external rotation of both feet. There is equal knee flexion/extension in order to prevent any sidebending of the lumbar spine. Right and left discrepancies in elevation (superior height) of anatomical landmarks are examined to assess coronal plane postural dysfunction. Right and left gluteal folds, PSIS, iliac crests, scapulae, shoulder girdles, ears, and eyes should all be on equal levels.

If the iliac crest is elevated on the right side compared to the left, there is a *pelvic obliquity*, which would contribute to a side bending (and rotation) of the lumbosacral spine. This could also contribute to functional leg length discrepancy. If the left shoulder girdle were elevated compared to the right, there would be a natural lateral shift of the lower cervical spine to the right. This would be similar to right cervical spine side bent posture. According to Fryettes' third law, left side bending would be limited in range of motion. If the patient compensates and presents with an elevated left shoulder girdle and a relatively straight neck, then the cervical spine is being maintained in left side bending, and there will be a limitation in right side bending. A pelvic girdle obliquity indicates limitations in lumbar range of motion. A right elevated iliac crest indicates that the lumbar spine is side bent to the right (up the kinetic chain), and there will be limitations in left lumbar side bending. A shoulder girdle obliquity indicates limitations in cervical ranges of motion. The cervical spine tends to compensate in order to maintain cranial balance in order to facilitate normal equilibrium and righting reactions of the brain stem.

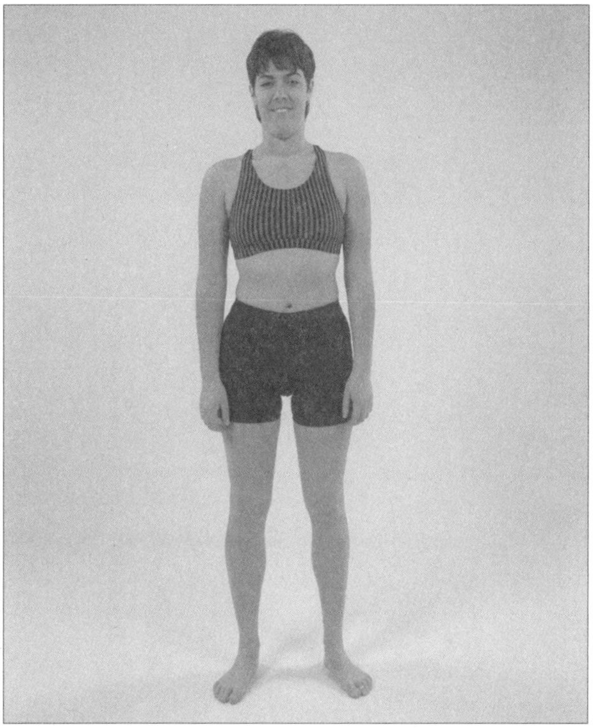

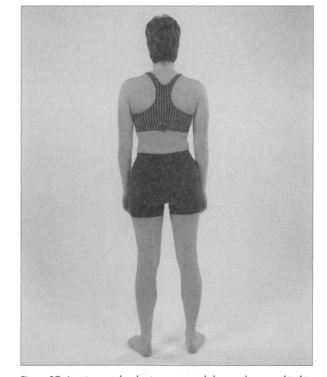

Figure 96. A static postural evaluation on a coronal plane can be assessed in this anterior standing view.

Figure 97. A static postural evaluation on a coronal plane can be assessed in this posterior standing view.

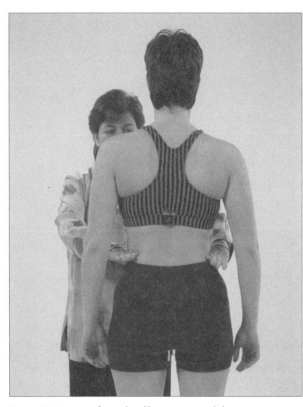

Figure 98. Assessment for a pelvic obliquity on a coronal plane.

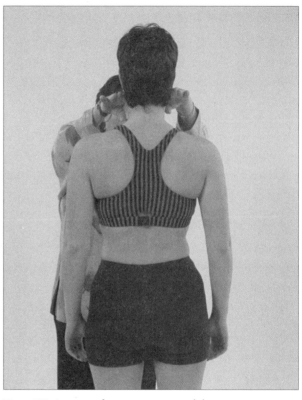

Figure 100. Assessment of ear position on a coronal plane.

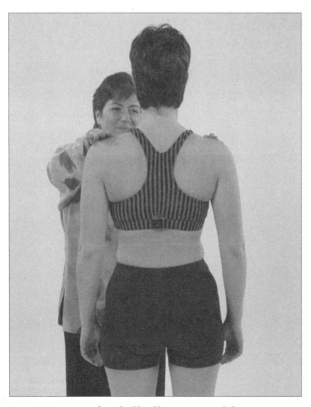

Figure 99. Assessment for a shoulder obliquity on a coronal plane.

Movement Assessment on a Coronal Plane

Static postural deviation can be interpreted to indicate physiologic limitations in ranges of motion. If there is a right pelvic obliquity and a resultant right side bending of the lumbar and lumbosacral spine, there may be full right side bending of the lumbar spine, but there cannot be full left lumbar side bending. If there is a left shoulder girdle obliquity, there will often be a compensatory deviation of the cervical spine to the right with limitations in side bending of the cervical spine. According to Fryette's third law of biomechanics, as we have seen, coronal plane postural dysfunction will correlate with limitations in range of motion on a sagittal plane and a transverse plane as well. Side bending will always be limited to one side. With an anterior view, there will be a right/left discrepancy of nipple lines and ASIS, as well as other anatomic landmarks.

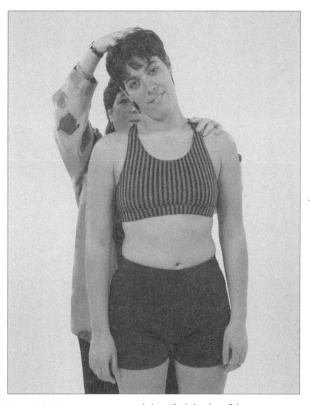

Figure 101. Assessment on a coronal plane of side bending of the spine.

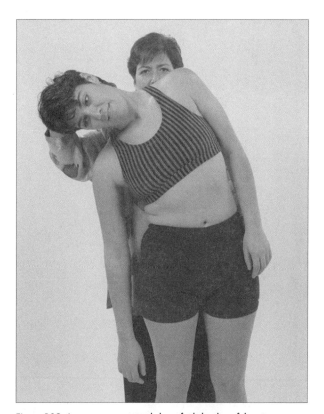

Figure 102. Assessment on a coronal plane of side bending of the spine.

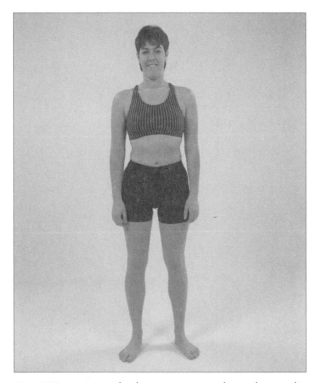

Figure 103. A static postural evaluation on a transverse plane can be assessed in this anterior standing view.

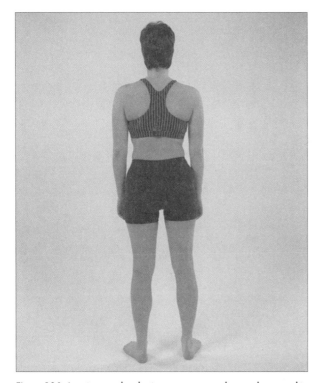

Figure 104. A static postural evaluation on a transverse plane can be assessed in this posterior standing view.

Transverse Plane Posture

Assessment on a coronal plane of side bending of the spine. Transverse plane postural dysfunction represents rotation dysfunction of the spine. The patient should stand with feet acetabular distance apart with feet equally externally rotated, and knees in an equally flexed/extended position. (See Figures 103 and 104.)

The transverse plane dysfunction can be assessed via assessment of the posterior prominence of the paravertebral soft tissue and transverse processes. The practitioner's fingers are lightly placed on both sides of the spine, over the paravertebral muscles. The hand, which is more prominent posteriorly, reflects rotation of those vertebrae to that side. The total spine, including cervical, thoracic, lumbar and sacral segments, can be evaluated for transverse plane postural asymmetry. If the right transverse processes are prominent posteriorly from T4 through T8, this represents a rotation dysfunction of the vertebrae T4 through T8 to the right with a limitation in left rotation of those segments. If the lumbar transverse processes and buttocks on the left are prominent posteriorly, this represents a transverse plane rotation dysfunction of L1 through the sacrum to the left with a limitation in right rotation of the lumbosacral spine.

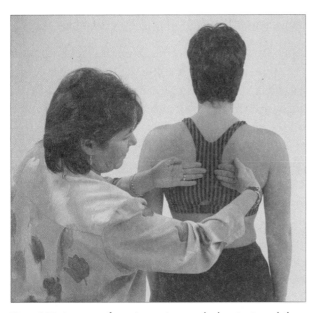

Figure 105. Assessment of posterior prominence at the thoracic spine and rib cage.

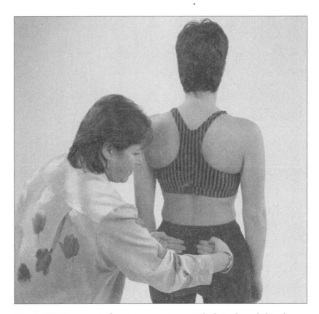

Figure 107 Assessment of posterior prominence at the buttocks and gluteal muscles.

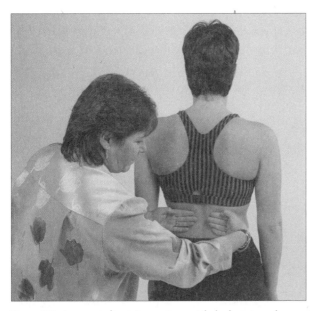

Figure 106. Assessment of posterior prominence at the lumbar spine and paravertebral musculature.

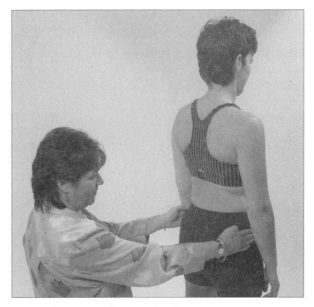

Figure 108. Assessment of rotation at the pelvis.

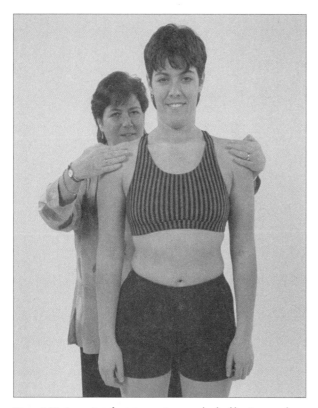

Figure 109. Assessment of anterior prominence at the shoulders (protracted shoulder girdles).

Movement Assessment of a Transverse Plane

Assessment on a coronal plane of sidebending of the spine. If there is a static postural deviation on a transverse plane, the therapist can anticipate finding limitation of motion in rotation to the opposite side. If T4 through T8 are stuck rotated to the right, there will be a limitation in left rotation of T4 through T8. Fryette's first law of biomechanics states that in neutral, rotation and side bending of the thoracic and lumbar spine occur to the opposite sides. If T4 through T8 are stuck in right rotation, they are also stuck in left side bending. These segments, from T4 through T8, will be limited in right side bending as well as left rotation.

There will be correlating information between posterior and anterior views during assessment of transverse plane dysfunction. (See Figure 109.) If T4 through T8 is prominent posteriorly on the right, the chest at this level will be prominent anteriorly on the left. Differentiation of transverse plane dysfunction of the spine from rib cage and shoulder girdle dysfunction is important.

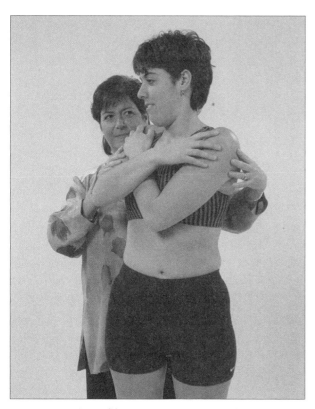

Figure 110. Assessment of thoracic rotation on a transverse plane.

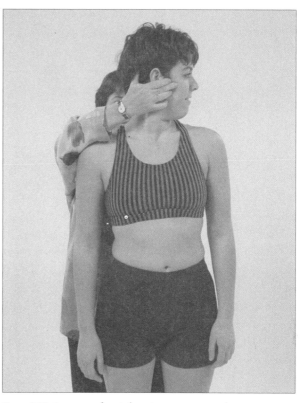

Figure 112. Assessment of cervical rotation on a transverse plane.

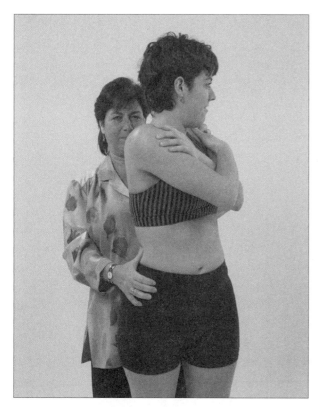

Figure 111. Assessment of thoracic rotation on a transverse plane.

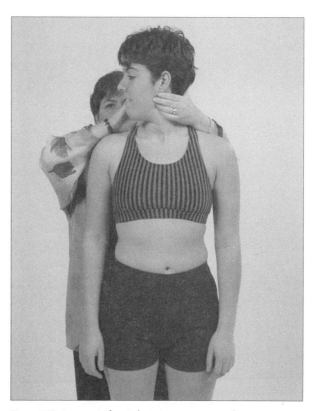

Figure 113. Assessment of cervical rotation on a transverse plane.

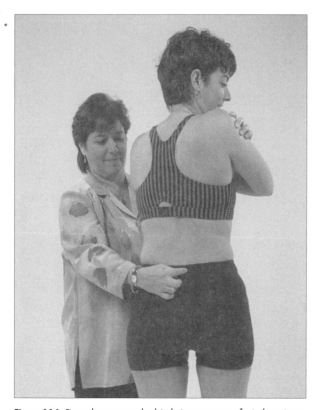

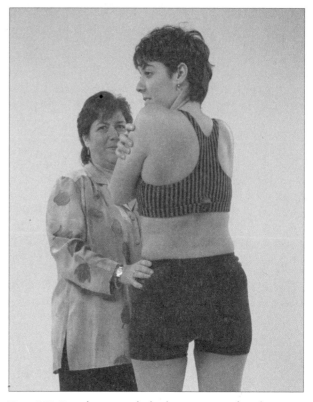

Figure 114. Fixate the sacrum and pelvis during assessment of spinal rotation to view uncompensated range of motion of the spine on a transverse plane.

Figure 115. Fixate the sacrum and pelvis during assessment of spinal rotation to view uncompensated range of motion of the spine on a transverse plane.

Postural Evaluation of the Extremities

The extremities can be evaluated for static and dynamic postural dysfunction on a sagittal, coronal, and transverse plane. For example, a protracted shoulder girdle is a static postural dysfunction on a transverse plane. On a dynamic postural assessment, because the right shoulder girdle is protracted, there may be full horizontal adduction, but there cannot be full horizontal abduction, because that should girdled cannot retract.

Upper Extremity

In order to attain *apparent* full physiologic range of motion, the body is capable of performing involuntary "trick" and compensatory movements to successfully achieve the desired horizontal abduction, or full extension, of the shoulder joint on the side. In order to attain this apparent physiologic range of motion, the humeral head will typically deviate from mid line during movement, in a compensatory attempt to attain the movement goals. The typical compensatory deviation of the humeral head is a tendency to sublux anteriorly within the glenoid fossa.

There are typical compensatory movements discovered during upper extremity dynamic postural (movement) evaluation (See Figures 116 and 117.) If there is a limitation in elbow extension and forearm supination, the proximal radial head will tend to shear anteriorly; the proximal ulnar head will abduct causing a medial gap; the distal ulnar head will shear anteriorly; the distal radial head will posteriorly shear; the proximal carpal row will shear anteriorly; the proximal first metacarpal head will deviate anteriorly and distally. *For normal pain-free movement, good articular balance without deviation or shears must be maintained throughout the physiologic ranges of motion.* The true limitation in joint mobility will then be noticeable. These compensatory deviations from midline during movement further exacerbate a hypomobile and painful neuromusculoskeletal condition.

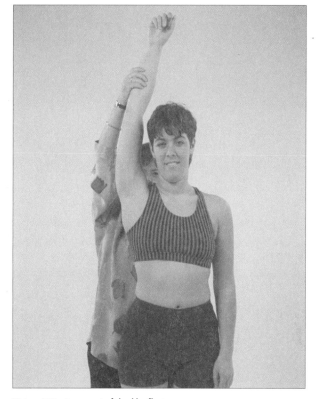

Figure 116. Assessment of shoulder flexion.

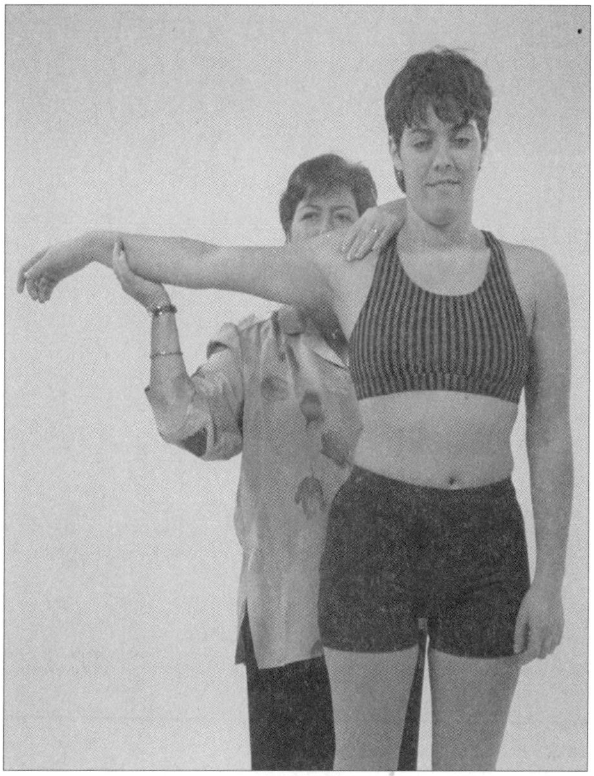

Figure 117. Assessment of shoulder horizontal abduction.

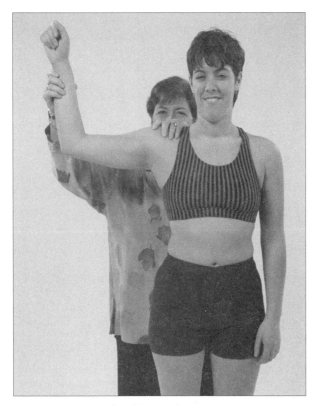

Figure 118. Assessment of shoulder external rotation.

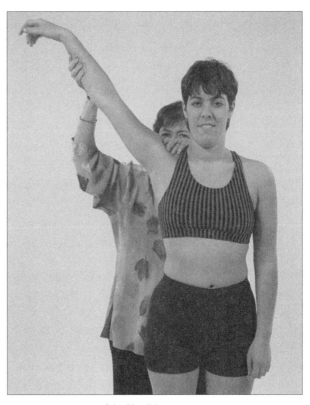

Figure 120. Assessment of shoulder abduction.

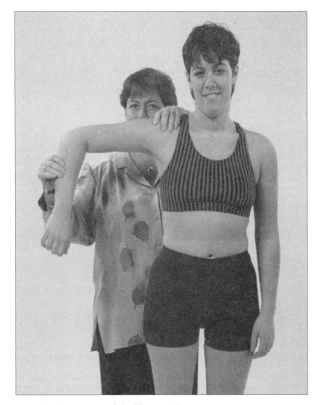

Figure 119. Assessment of shoulder internal rotation.

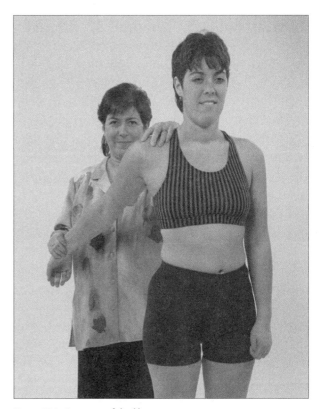

Figure 121. Assessment of shoulder extension.

Lower Extremity

Typical hip joint dysfunction includes an approximated, adducted, internally rotated and inferiorly displaced femoral head within the acetabulum. In the standing and in the recumbent position, this approximation of hip joint surfaces may be palpated by placing the hands over the *greater trochanter.*

Knee joint dysfunction typically presents with an externally rotated and laterally sheared proximal tibial articular surface.

Ankle joint dysfunction, which includes the *tibiotalar* and *subtalar* joints, typically present with a posterior shear of tibia on talus, an inferior lateral *malleolus*, an inverted *calcaneus*, and intra-articular adhesions of the talo-calcaneal joint. Supinated (high arch) and pronated (flat foot) postural deviations of the feet are common.

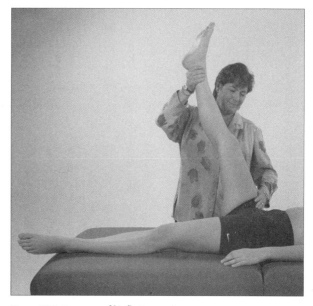

Figure 122. Assessment of hip flexion.

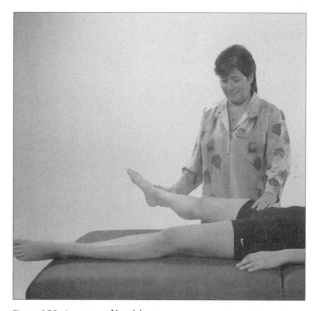

Figure 123. Assessment of hip abduction.

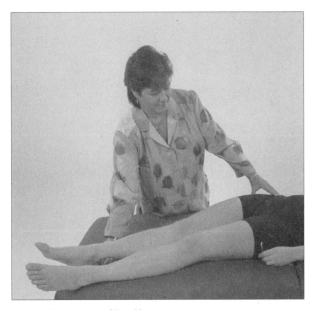

Figure 124. Assessment of hip adduction.

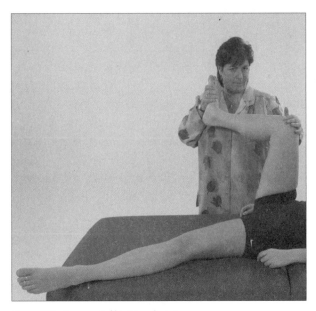

Figure 126. Assessment of hip internal rotation.

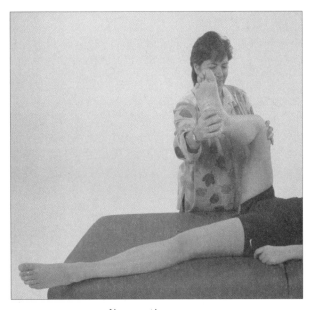

Figure 125. Assessment of hip external rotation.

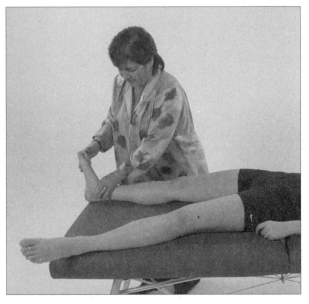

Figure 127. Assessment of ankle dorsiflexion.

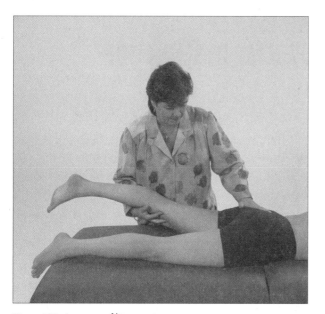

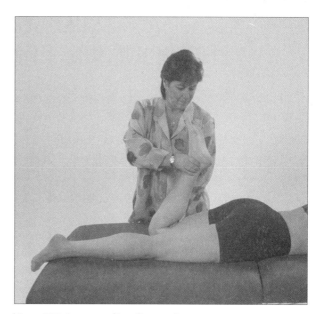

Figure 128. Assessment of hip extension.

Figure 129. Assessment of knee flexion and extension.

CHAPTER 23

FASCIAL GLIDE ASSESSMENT FOR INDICATIONS OF MYOFASCIAL DYSFUNCTION

The connective tissue system is a continuous, contiguous system, which envelops every cell and fiber in the body and is the immediate environment for every cell. Fascial dysfunction within the connective tissue system, and other neuromusculoskeletal dysfunction, are reflected in the fascia.

Evaluation of fascial glide can assess the mobility and flexibility of the connective tissue system: is the soft tissue mobile and friction-free during movement? The practitioner's hands are gently but firmly placed on the body. The practitioner can begin by standing at the patient's feet with a hand on each leg, while the patient is in a supine position. The practitioner can assess the fascial glide throughout the anterior surface of the body. Upon completion, the fascial glide evaluation process is repeated with the patient in a prone position. Three layers of fascial glide can be assessed: (1) skin on superficial fascia; (2) deeper fascial restrictions; (3) deepest soft tissue mobility: soft tissue on bone.

The practitioner is palpating tissue mobility, flexibility, and freedom of tissue glide. If the fascial glide appears compromised, tight, hypomobile, or inflexible, the therapist can document this on a body diagram as indication for Fascial Release.

Manual Therapy for treatment of dysfunction of the connective tissue system is Myofascial Release. Myofascial Release can be performed at the areas documented on the body diagram. Soft tissue myofascial releases as described in the text can be performed in all areas of decreased and compromised Fascial Glide and positive Myofascial Mapping. Articular Fascial releases as described in this text can be performed after soft tissue myofascial release at the joint surfaces, where Myofascial Mapping and Fascial Glide present positive findings.

Fascial Glide

The practitioner's hands assess the mobility of the fascial tissue on three planes.

1. The hands glide the soft tissue superiorly and then glide the soft tissue inferiorly, to assess freedom of tissue mobility in those directions.
2. The hands then glide the tissue medially and then laterally.
3. The hands next glide the tissue clockwise and then counterclockwise.

CHAPTER 24

MYOFASCIAL MAPPING

Theory of Myofascial Dysfunction: Hypothetical Model Related to the Phenomenon of Myofascial Mapping

Myofascial dysfunction is the problematic process that occurs within the ground substance, the fibers, cells, and other substances and energetic components of the connective tissue.

All of the soft tissues are affected in anatomic areas where myofascial dysfunction is present. Since the substance of the connective tissue envelops and infiltrates at the level of the sarcomere, it is more correct to use the term *myofascial dysfunction* rather than *fascial* dysfunction, but the term "myofascial dysfunction" is not always correct terminology to reflect the disorder. The primary pathology is within the connective tissue (fascial) system; the muscle fiber tissue is affected as a secondary problem.

Connective tissue encompasses many tissues and structures including bone, fascial envelopes, nerves, blood cells, and other tissue. These tissues and structures all have the potential to be affected with myofascial dysfunction. That means, a bone may be determined to have myofascial dysfunction as may a circulatory vessel or a neuron.

Sharon (Weiselfish) Giammatteo discovered Myofascial Mapping. Myofascial Mapping (MFMapping) is the practice of differential diagnosis via evidence that the fascial motility has been affected. Motility is the inherent rhythmic cycle of the physiologic pressure affecting a tissue, structure, system, or other aspect of the body's anatomy. Motility is a circadian rhythm, a universal presentation that manifests in a manner unique to the physiologically characteristic traits of that anatomy.

The term Myofascial Mapping refers both to a diagnostic task and physologic motility. As a *motility*, it is the biological rhythm of the connective tissue. When a practitioner performs the *task* of Myofascial Mapping in a given area, he or she is palpating the rhythm of the fascia and looking for a distortion in that area. When performing Myofascial Mapping, one documents the areas of distortion on a body diagram.

The task of Myofascial Mapping is a procedure that discovers the motility of the ground substance in the connective tissue. The flagellae of the glycosaminoglycans (GAGs) are apparently responsible for the unique characteristic traits of MFMapping. Their inherent motion, which is rhythmic and cyclical, is dependent upon the physiologic and energetic conditions of the region. Occasionally, the total body rhythm (MFMapping) is affected because an organ of significance is extremely dysfunctional, affecting all the flagellae of all the GAGs in the body. This positive, total body MFMapping phenomenon indicates a need for medical investigation before there is a breakdown of an organ's function.

When assessing MFMapping, there are three possibilities: (1) Positive mapping: an asymmetric motion of the fascial tissue; (2) negative mapping: a symmetric motions of the fascial tissue; and (3) *still space:* no evident motion of the fascial tissue.

The three planes of mapping are transverse, sagittal, and coronal. Internal rotation and external rotation are the motions of the fascial tissue on the transverse plane. Flexion and extension are the motions of the fascial tissue on the sagittal plane. Abduction and adduction are the motions of the fascial tissue on the coronal plane. All of the motions on the transverse, sagittal, and coronal planes are reflected on the body. When the hands of the therapist are in body contact, these motions of internal rotation, external rotation, flexions, extension, abduction, and adduction can be discerned.

Experimental clinical research has indicated evidence on three levels: Level One MFMapping reflects the body's neuromusculoskeletal function and dysfunction. This can be confirmed with MFMapping on the body's surface. Level Two MFMapping reflects emotional, energetic body function and dysfunction. Level Three MFMapping reflects the cognitive/mental energetic function and dysfunction, as well as spiritual/other energetic function and dysfunction that may be affecting the body.

Unique qualities of MFMapping are associated with Levels One, Two, and Three. Level One will reflect the physical body's dysfunction manifesting through transverse plane internal rotation and external rotation. Other planes of MFMapping, including coronal plane (abduction and adduction), and sagittal plane (flexion and extension) are not discovered on Level One. Level Two will reflect the emotional energy dysfunction with transverse plane motion (internal rotation and external rotation). Level Two will not provide any indication of coronal plane and sagittal plane motions. On Level Three, there is a reflection of: (1) mental/cognitive energies discovered on a coronal plane as abduction and adduction; and (2) spiritual/other energies discerned on a sagittal plane as flexion and extension. Transverse plane motions of internal rotation and external rotation are not evident on Level Three.

The motions possible with MFMapping are: (1) symmetric; (2) asymmetric; (3) no motion. Symmetric motions indicate healthy and functional fascial motilities. Asymmetric motions indicate unhealthy and dysfunctional fascial motilities. Still space (no motion), which can only be palpated on a transverse plane, indicates the pathologic pressures of other energies (emotional/mental/cognitive, spiritual/other) affecting the fascial motilities.

The motions are palpated in the following manner. Place hands next to each other (smaller areas can be palpated with just the fingers). Then rest hands lightly (like a feather) on the body's surface (and off the body for palpation of the three levels). Let the body's tissues move the hands. Both hands may be moved in the same direction (symmetric motion), or in opposite directions (asymmetric motion). The hands may remain still (no movement).

When the motion is symmetric, the MFMapping is termed *Negative Mapping.* When the motion is asymmetric, the MFMapping is termed *Positive Mapping.* Where there is no motion, the MFMapping term is *Still Space.* (Still spaces are only palpated on a transverse plane, as we mentioned before.)

The inherent motility of the flagellae of the glycosaminoglycans is peculiar to the metabolic cycle. Metabolism has many characteristics, one of which is an inhalation and exhalation cycle ((Weiselfish) Giammatteo) of the metabolic transport of nutrients and waste products into and out of the cells. During the inhalation phase the nutrients enter the cell and waste products are excreted from it. During the exhalation phase there is a reorganization of the flagellae in preparation for the next inhalation phase. The inhalation phase is the more active, opening phase of the metabolic cycle. The exhalation phase is the more passive, closed phase of the cycle. Because the MFMapping reflects the metabolic cycle of inhalation phase and exhalation phase, there are characteristic motions for each. The motions of fascial motility of the inhalation phase include flexion, adduction, and internal rotation. The motions of the exhalation phase are extension, adduction, and external rotation.

There is no single or unique frequency of fascial motility reflected with MFMapping. The organized, healthy, and functional motility will vary from 5 to 15 cycles per minute. This means, one cycle includes the flexion, adduction, internal rotation of the inhalation phase plus the extension, abduction, external rotation of the exhalation phase. A rhythm of lower frequency may reflect sluggish metabolism. A rhythm of higher frequency may reflect hyperactive metabolism. There is a wide range for normal fascial motility and there are several hypothetical explanations for the variability. In Eastern medicine, the rhythmic rate can indicate which "element" (wood, fire, earth, metal, or water) is most powerful in that person. In Western medicine, it can indicate whether a person possesses an *endomorphic, ectomorphic,* or *mesomorphic* structure.

MFMapping will reflect whatever tissue or structure is in dysfunction and therefore is affecting fascial motility. If a bone is fractured, for example, the frequency is quick (greater than 15 cycles per minute) and there will be a sharp interphase (between inhalation phase and exhalation phase). When a muscle is ruptured or hurt, the frequency is slow (less than 5 cycles per minute) with a sluggish interphase. When an organ is compromised (whether or not anatomic dysfunction is already reflected by physiologic changes), the frequency will be normal (within 5 to 15 cycles per minutes), but a very wide amplitude of fascia motility will be evident, and the interphase will be acute. When the nervous tissues are compromised, whether there is neural tension, brain or spinal cord fibrosis, nerve root impingement, or other problems of the central and peripheral nervous tissue, the MFMapping will have small amplitude, high frequency, and a mild interphase. It is anticipated that future research will provide further clarity regarding these rhythms to assist in differential diagnosis.

An Overview of the Clinical Practice of Myofascial Mapping

Myofascial Mapping is a practice for the differential diagnosis of neuromusculoskeletal dysfunction.

Three MFMapping outcomes, as we mentioned above, are possible: positive mapping, negative mapping; and Still Space. Positive mapping

in a given area indicates neuromusculoskeletal dysfunction. The dysfunctional tissue or structure could be bone, blood vessel, muscle fiber, connective tissue cells or fibers, ground substance, organs, nerves; or other tissues and structures. In the area of negative MFMapping, there is no indication of neuromusculoskeletal dysfunction. A Still Space, which is only palpated on a transverse plane, is an area where there is neither positive nor negative mapping. What we refer to as "other energies" produce the Still Space.

Negative MFMapping reflects the active symmetric, rhythmical movement of the body's tissues, which we suggest is a result of the cyclic and rhythmical movement of the flagellae of the glycosaminoglycans of the connective tissue. This active, symmetric rhythm is a reflection of the perfusion of healthy energy and the entropy of normal tissue. When there is a negative MFMapping, the tissue is actively moving in a symmetric manner on all three planes in alternating phases. There is a phase of inhalation and a cycle of exhalation as we mentioned above. Internal rotation occurs on the transverse plane during the inhalation cycle; external rotation occurs on the transverse plane during the exhalation cycle.

Inhalation Cycle and Exhalation Cycle

The cycles of inhalation and exhalation do not refer to the respiratory movement. These terms refer to intake capacity (inhalation) and exit capacity (exhalation) within the ground substance of the connective tissue. During the inhalation cycle, the ground substance distributes nutrients to the cells and takes in waste products exiting from the cells. During the exhalation cycle, the ground substance realigns its protein, especially the glycosaminoglycans (GAGs), in order to prepare for the active metabolic process that occurs during the inhalation cycle.

When MFMapping is positive on one or more planes, there is an active, asymmetric, asynchronous, cyclical movement of the tissues that reflects a region of dysfunctional inhalation and exhalation process within the connective tissue. On either side of the area of dysfunction, and within that area, internal rotation will occur at the same time as external rotation if the dysfunction is on a transverse plane. Adduction will occur at the same time as abduction if it is on a coronal plane. Flexion will occur together with extension if it is on a sagittal plane. This asymmetric activity reflects an inability of the tissues in that region to respond effectively and efficiently to the metabolic process. This asynchrony of the inhalation and exhalation cycles indicates tissue dysfunction that is disrupting the motility of glycosaminoglycans. This loss of symmetrical movement is a reflection of tissue disorder, which may be primary and/or secondary, or in the GAGs of the ground substance. Every dysfunction in the body can affect this aspect of the ground substance. The ground substance is the environment for every cell, fiber, organ, structure, and system.

When MFMapping on a transverse plane is a Still Space, this indicates that there is an energetic disturbance influencing the motility of the GAGs. This energy may be emotional energy, mental/cognitive energy, or spiritual and /or other energy.

When more than one energy (i.e., emotional, mental/cognitive, spiritual/other) affects the ground substance, there are pressure changes that occur which cause a profound Still Space. These pressure changes occur whenever emotional energy intersects with mental/cognitive energy and/or spiritual/other energy. These pathologic pressures cause a quieting of the motility of the flagellae of the glycosaminoglycans; they do not practice in their normal fashion. When there is a Still Space, the inhalation and exhalation cycle within the tissues are shut down. There is a compromise of metabolism within this region as a result.

The clinical phenomenon which occurs in the tissue when two or more of these energies intersect, causing a still space, is similar to the effect of dropping a pebble in a clear pool of water; ripple effects of energy distribute, radiating from all points around that spot. Waves of energy are emitted from the space of intersection of energies.

John Upledger, D.O., first described this clinical phenomenon of a pebble dropped into a clear pool of water and the resultant energetic disturbance, perceived as a ripple effect. He calls this phenomenon *"arcing."* Arcing can isolate primary areas in the body that require treatment. These are areas that more profoundly affecting the person. There is an emotional and/or mental/cognitive and/or spiritual/other component involved in that person's process. Two (or more) of these energies must be affecting the tissue in order for them to intersect. This intersection of energies causes the pressure changes that result in the phenomenon of arcing discovered by Dr. Upledger. Thus, arcing is a tool for differential diagnosis, to be used to discover in which areas of the body there is metabolic process, involving an emotional, mental/cognitive, spiritual/other component.

Jean Pierre Barral, D.O. discovered and documented three planes of energy that can be palpated above the body. The first plane lies 8 cm off the body in the supine and the prone position. The second plane lies 12 cm off the body. The third plane is found approximately 18 cm off the body. Barral states that the first plane energy reflects the status of the physical body. Areas of increased heat on this plane indicate neuromusculoskeletal dysfunction. The second plane reflects the emotional status of the body. Areas of dysfunction are reflected on the first and second planes as increased heat. Barral and his colleagues in France developed equipment that can discern increases of heat on these two planes. Barral received an award from the French Government for this equipment.

MFMapping can also be performed on the first and second planes. In the context of MFMapping, these planes are referred to as "levels of reference." On the first level, where physical neuromusculoskeletal dysfunction is manifested, mapping can be positive on a transverse plane, a coronal plane, and a sagittal plane.

The still space can also be palpated on the first level. When the still space is discerned on a transverse plane, this is a reflection of emotional energy disturbing the tissues.

On the second level (12 cm off the body), the MFMapping will be positive only on a transverse plane. This plane only reflects a disturbance of emotional energy. Mental/cognitive, spiritual/other, and physical neuromusculoskeletal dysfunction will not be reflected on the second level.

On the third level (approximately 18 cm off the body) energetic disturbance and neuromusculoskeletal fascial dysfunction can be palpated on the coronal and sagittal planes. The coronal plane at this level indicates mental/cognitive energy. When the mapping is evident on the sagittal plane at this level, it reflects that spiritual/other energy is affecting the ground substance.

Local Listening and *Referred Listening* are further differential diagnostic techniques developed by Barral. They are performed by putting one's hands over the patient's body and paying attention to fascial restrictions and tensions as if one were listening with one's hands. They can be performed on all three levels and between levels to help in discovering the dominant and primary problems.

In general, MFMapping can be performed on the body, on all three levels. The findings are documented on a body diagram showing all vies: anterior, posterior, right lateral, left lateral. Local Listening and Referred Listening can then be performed in order to find associated problems, as well as to identify the more dominant and more primary problems.

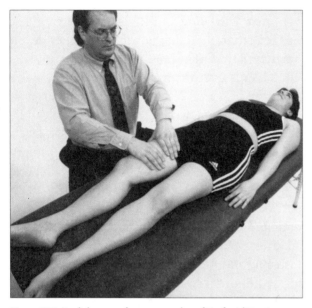

Figure 130. Hand placements for transverse plane of Myofascial Mapping.

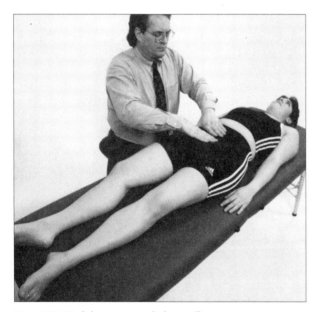

Figure 131. Hand placement perpendicular to midline.

The Application of Myofascial Mapping

In performing MFMapping, the hands are placed side by side on the bare body's surface. It is easier to palpate over skin than over clothes. The hands are "feather-light," so that no real weight is actually pressing on the body. The hands are relaxed, without tension, and are able to be moved by the very slight force of fascial motion.

These photos depict the appropriate hand position for Myofascial Mapping. To palpate the transverse plane rhythm, place your hands perpendicular to midline.

1. When the hands are moved together in the same direction, the MFMapping is negative. This means that there is no evidence of neuromusculoskeletal dysfunction.

2. When the hands are moved in opposite directions at the same time, the MFMapping is *positive*. This means that there is evidence of neuromusculoskeletal dysfunction.

3. When the hands are resting lightly on the body on a transverse plane, but the hands are not moved (i.e., there is no fascial motility exerting a force on the tissues in any direction), the MFMapping is a *Still Space*. This means there is evidence of emotional energies affecting the neuromusculoskeletal fascial tissues and structures.

It is common practice to perform total body MFMapping at an initial evaluation session. This is performed on the anterior, lateral, and posterior surfaces of the body (total body surface). Common practice is to start at the feet and progress to the head, doing MFMapping on the anterior surface (in supine position) first. It is possible to find MFMapping positive at very small body areas (e.g., a toe, over a joint, over a ligament) and over very large body areas (e.g., a limb, a lung/rib cage, low back). Still Spaces are usually found over smaller areas on a transverse plane and are commonly discerned at the anterior neck, the frontals, the heart, kidneys, the pelvic region, and other areas that have been found significant for holding emotional energies.

When MFMapping is performed on the body it is possible to find:

1. Negative mapping on a transverse plane.
2. Negative napping on a coronal plane.
3. Negative mapping on a sagittal plane.
4. Positive mapping on a transverse plane.
5. Positive mapping on a coronal plane.
6. Positive mapping on a sagittal plane.
7. Still space on a transverse plane.

When MF Mapping is performed approximately 4 inches off the body on Level One, it is possible to find:

1. Positive mapping on a transverse plane
2. Negative mapping on a transverse plane
3. Still space on a transverse plane.

MFMapping on Level One, approximately 4 inches off the body, reflects only physical neuromusculoskeletal dysfunction.

When MF Mapping is performed approximately eight inches off the body on Level Two, it is possible to find:

1. Positive mapping on a transverse plane
2. Negative napping on a transverse plane.

MFMapping on Level Two reflects the emotional energy that is contributing to fascial dysfunction and affecting neuromusculoskeletal dysfunction.

When MFMapping is performed approximately 12 inches off the body on Level Three, it is possible to find:

1. Positive mapping on a coronal plane.
2. Negative mapping on a coronal plane.
3. Positive mapping on a sagittal plane.
4. Negative mapping on a sagittal plane.

Coronal Plane MFMapping can be palpated approximately twelve inches off the body on Level Three and reflects the mental/cognitive energies that are influencing fascial motility and affecting neuromusculoskeletal function. Sagittal Plane MFMapping can be palpated approximately twelve inches off the body on Level Three and reflects the spiritual/other energies that are influencing fascial motility and affecting neuromusculoskeletal function.

When MFMapping is performed on a transverse plane, the hands are placed in a medial/lateral direction, palms facing the body surface. When MFMapping is performed on a coronal plane or on a sagittal plane, the hands are placed in a superior/inferior direction, palms facing the body surface.

Occasionally, the Still Space discovered via MFMapping is more "profound" than usual: there is a perception on palpation that all of the rhythms (fascial motilities, craniosacral rhythm, arterial pulse, venous flow, pulmonary rhythm) are compromised. These areas have at least two or more planes of MFMapping showing positive on a sagittal, coronal, or one of these plus a still space on a transverse plane.

Positive MFMapping will be present on Level Two and/or Level Three. Level One will have an aspect of emotional energy, while Level Three will have an aspect of mental/cognitive energies and/or spiritual/other energies affecting fascial motility. When two energies meet and intersect, there is an apparent pressure change at the point of intersection. Energies will radiate in a circle from that point. John Upledger, D.O. has dubbed the clinical phenomena of these energies radiating from the intersection point as "arcing" as we mentioned above. He discovered that arcing indicates both profound and primary areas of body problems, which must be addressed for effective and efficient recovery.

General Listening, Local Listening, and Referred Listening are diagnostic techniques developed by Jean Pierre Barral, D.O. General Listening allows the practitioner to discover the areas of mechanical tension in the body that affect posture, soft tissue, and joint mobility. At the time of assessment, General Listening will reveal a region to be treated. MFMapping can then indicate the specific tissues/structures that are dysfunctional within that area.

Local Listening allows the practitioner to discover areas of dysfunction that are related to other areas of dysfunction which have already been discovered. MFMapping will further discern which of these related areas are primary areas of neuromusculoskeletal dysfunction. Local Listening can discern which tissue is primary and dominant over others.

Referred Listening discovers different areas of the body with similar associated pressures affecting the tissues. MFMapping can further distinguish if these areas present a primary dysfunction or only a secondary one as the result of dysfunction at another location.

Paul Chauffour, D.O., developed Inhibitory Balance Testing to discover a patient's most dominant neuromusculoskeletofascial dysfunction. MFMapping will reflect a primary dysfunction at sites discovered with Inhibitory Balance Testing.

It is possible to distinguish which Level (Body, One, Two, or Three) has the primary, dominant problem. With Local Listening, the *dominant* region of MFMapping can be discovered as well as which level is contributing more to the production of signs and symptoms. Referred Listening can be performed on all Levels (Body, One, Two, Three) so that the *primary* level of significance can be discovered.

PART FIVE

PROTOCOLS

CHAPTER 25

THE BASIC PROTOCOLS OF MYOFASCIAL RELEASE

How to Use this Chapter

This part of the book includes protocols (listed alphabetically) for effective and efficient application particularly valuable for the beginner. Once you have grasped the concept of addressing the pathoanatomic site of dysfunction with the Myofascial Release 3-Planar Fascial Fulcrum Approach and you are comfortable with the technique you do not need to limit yourself strictly to the methods of this approach.

Read the protocols. Look at the techniques outlined in Part Four of this book. Follow the recommended sequences. These sequences are the result of almost fifteen years of research and have been designed to assure client satisfaction, improved functional outcome, increased efficiency, and decreased treatment reaction and side effects.

Occiasionally, you will find mention of techniques not developed in this book. You will find them in early volumes of *Integrative Manual Therapy*.

Abdominal Cramps

TREATMENT

1. The Spinal Protocol (Steps 1 to 14.)

2. Respiratory System Protocol (Steps 1 to 7.)

   ▪ All symmetric ganglia must be decompressed from the costovertebral joints.

3. Cranio-cervical junction

   ▪ The vagus nerve (cranial nerve X) must be decompressed in the suboccipital space.

4. Soft Tissue Myofascial Release Technique

   ▪ Perform this technique with an anterior/posterior hold over the cardiac sphincter (hiatus between oesophagus and stomach).

   ▪ The vagus nerve is often compromised at the cardiac sphincter.

5. Soft Tissue Myofascial Release Technique

   ▪ Perform this technique with anterior/posterior holds for each of the four abdominal quadrants (right upper, left upper, right lower, left lower).

   ▪ Perform 4 repetitions of this technique.

6. Articular Myofascial Release: anterior and posterior iliosacral joints

   ▪ This is a technique from the Spinal Protocol that is repeated here.

7. Soft Tissue and Articular Fascial Release: thoracolumbar junction

   ▪ This is a technique from the Spinal Protocol that is repeated here.

8. Soft Tissue Myofascial Releases: transverse diaphragms (pelvic, respiratory abdominal, thoracic inlet).

   ▪ This is a technique from the Spinal Protocol that is repeated here.

Anterior Compartment Syndrome

TREATMENT

1. The Spinal Protocol (Steps 1 to 14.) should be considered.

2. Cervical Syndrome and Neck Pain Protocol (Steps 1 to 3.)

3. Shoulder Joint Dysfunction Protocol (Steps 1 to 5.)

   ▪ Almost all cases of anterior compartment syndrome are double crush phenomena.

4. Soft Tissue Myofascial Release Technique: forearm

5. Hanging Technique: Radioulnar Joint

   ▪ Repeat. (This technique was performed in Step 3.)

6. Soft Tissue Myofascial Release Technique: wrist joint

Cervical Syndrome and Neck Pain

TREATMENT

1. The Spinal Protocol (Steps 1 to 14.)
2. Soft Tissue Myofascial Release Technique: lateral neck hold
   - If the Scalenes Compression Test for brachial plexus compression is positive, repeat this technique 2 to 5 times. Repeat the Scalenes Compression Test after each repetition until the findings are negative.
   - When there is neurologic dysfunction such as Erb's palsy, Klumpke's palsy, mixed palsy, torticollis, upper extremity spasticity (e.g., hemipelgia), repeat this techniques 2 to 5 times.
   - These techniques may achieve full bilateral cervical rotation and side bending.
3. Hyoid Technique: Four Phases
   - If there is dysphasia, status post tracheotomy, repeat these 4 phases 4 times each.
   - With facial and temporomandibular joint pain, repeat these 4 phases 2 times each.

Elbow Joint Problems

Including Tennis Elbow, Golfer's Elbow, and Ulnar Groove Compression

TREATMENT

1. The Spinal Protocol (Steps 1 to 14.) should be considered.
2. Cervical Syndrome and Neck Pain protocol (Steps 1 to 3.)
3. Shoulder Joint Dysfunction protocol (Steps 1 to 9.)
4. Soft Tissue Myofascial Release Technique: elbow joint
5. Articular Myofascial Release Technique: (a) radiohumeral joint; (b) humeroulnar joint
6. Hanging Technique: radioulnar joint
7. Muscle Belly Technique: (a) biceps; (b) triceps; (c) brachioradialis
8. Scar Tissue Release Technique: brachioradialis tendon
   - This technique is necessary for tennis elbow when there is a history of hydrocortisone injection.

Carpal Tunnel Syndrome

TREATMENT

1. The Spinal Protocol (Steps 1 to 4.) should be considered.
2. Cervical Syndrome and Neck Pain protocol (Steps 1 to 3.)
3. Shoulder Joint Dysfunction protocol (Steps 1 to 9.)
   - Almost all cases of carpal tunnel are double crush phenomena.
4. Soft Tissue Myofascial Release Techniques: wrist joints
5. Articular Myofascial Release Technique: wrist joints
6. Hanging Technique: radioulnar joint
7. Articular Myofascial Release Technique: first carpal metacarpal joint
8. Soft Tissue Myofascial Release Technique: hand
9. Retinaculum Technique: carpal retinaculum
10. Scar Tissue Release Technique: post-surgical carpal tunnel scars (wrist scars)
    - If EMG and NCV electrodiagnostic results remain positive, Neural Tissue Tension techniques can be performed.

Cerebral Palsy

TREATMENT

1. The Spinal Protocol (Steps 1 to 14.)
   - Repeat this protocol 5 to 10 times.
2. Cervical Syndrome and Neck Pain protocol: (Steps 1 to 3.)
3. Respiratory System protocol (Steps 1 to 7.)
   - Repeat this protocol 5 to 10 times.
4. Synergic Pattern Release protocol
   - (See *Integrative Manual Therapy for the Upper and Lower Extremities* by Sharon (Weiselfish) Giammatteo, Ph.D., P.T.)
   - Bilateral lower extremities (treat spastic side first).
5. Synergic Pattern Release protocol
   - (See *Integrative Manual Therapy for the Upper and Lower Extremities* by Sharon (Weiselfish) Giammatteo, Ph.D., P.T.)
   - Bilateral upper extremities (treat spastic side first).
6. Cranial therapy is indicated.

Chondromalacia

1. The Spinal Protocol (Steps 1 to 14.). All steps of this protocol should be considered.
2. Soft Tissue Myofascial Release Technique: knee joint
3. Soft Tissue Myofascial Release Technique: ankle joint
4. Soft Tissue Myofascial Release Technique: foot and plantar Fascia
5. Articular Fascial Release Technique: knee joint
6. Articular Fascial Release Technique: ankle joints (tibiotalar and subtalar)
   - Dorsiflexion must be restored to positive 10 degrees. When midstance is in plantar flexion rather than 0 degrees neutral, and midstance through toe off does not have anterior tibial glide over talus, then extensor forces are transcribed up the leg. These forces hit the posterior surface of the patella causing a defibrillation of the hyaline cartilage.
7. Hanging Technique: tibiofibular joint
8. Patellar Release (See page 106.)
9. Muscle Belly Technique: quadriceps, hamstrings, gastrocnemius

Erb's Palsy, Klumke's Palsy, Mixed Palsy

1. The Spinal Protocol (Steps 1 to 14.)
2. Cervical Syndrome and Neck Pain protocol
   - The Lateral Hold for the Soft Tissue Myofascial Release Technique may be repeated 5 to 10 times.
   - With Erb's palsy be sure to address the upper neck (C1 to C5). With Klumke's palsy be sure to address the lower neck (C5 to T1). With mixed palsy be sure to address the whole neck.
3. Shoulder Joint Dysfunction protocol
   - This needs to be repeated several times with Erb's palsy. It may not be necessary with Klumke's palsy.
4. Soft Tissue Myofascial Release Technique: elbow joint, forearm, wrist, hand, fingers
   - This needs to be repeated several times with Klumke's Palsy and mixed palsies. It may not be required with Erb's palsy.
5. Articular Fascial Release Technique: elbow joints (radiohumeral, ulnarhumeral)
   - This is required for Klumke's and mixed palsies. It may not be necessary for Erb's palsy.
6. Hanging Technique: radioulnar joint
7. Articular Myofascial Release Technique: wrist joints, metacarpal joints, metacarpal phalangeal joints, interphalangeal joints (all five digits).

Hand Dysfunction and Status Post Surgery

TREATMENT

1. The Spinal Protocol (Steps 1 to 14.) should be considered.

2. Cervical Syndrome and Neck Pain protocol (Steps 1 to 3.) should be considered.

3. Shoulder Joint Dysfunction protocol (Steps 1 to 5.) should be considered.

4. Soft Tissue Myofascial Release Technique: wrist joint

5. Articular Myofascial Release Technique: wrist joint

6. Retinaculum Technique: carpal tunnel, hand (palm), fingers

7. Soft Tissue Myofascial Release Technique: thumb and all fingers

9. Articular Myofascial Release Techniques: carpal joints, metacarpal joints, metacarpal phalangeal joint, interphalangeal joints of all five digits

10. Capsule and Ligament Techniques: thumb and fingers

Osteoarthritis (All Joints)

TREATMENT

1. The Spinal Protocol (Steps 1 to 14.)

2. Soft Tissue Myofascial Release Technique: All joints of the dysfunctional extremity

   • For example, osteoarthritis of the right knee joint will require Soft Tissue Myofascial Release technique over right hip, right knee, right ankle and right foot joints.

3. Articular Myofascial Release Technique: all joints of the dysfunctional extremity

   • For example, osteoarthritis of the right knee joint requires Articular Myofascial Release technique at the right hip joint, right tibiofibular joint, right tibiotalar joint, right subtalar joint; it also requires Hanging Technique for the right tibiofibular joint, all right tarsal, tarsal metatarsal, metatarsal phalangeal,and interphalangeal joints.

4. Articular Myofascial Release Technique

   • Perform this technique for the primary osteoarthritic joint. Repeat the technique 3 to 10 times, at 1 week intervals.

5. Muscle Belly Technique: all major muscles of the dysfunctional extremity

   • For example, osteoarthritis of the right knee joint requires the Muscle Belly Technique for the right hamstrings, right quadriceps, right gastrocnemius, right tibialis anterior, and right peroneals.

6. Ligament and Capsule Technique: of the primary osteoarthritic joint

Plantar Fascitis

1. The Spinal Protocol (Steps 1 to 14.)
2. Soft Tissue Myofascial Release Technique: all joints and soft tissues of the extremity, proximal to distal
3. Soft Tissue Myofascial Release Technique: ankle joints (tibiotalar and subtalar)
4. Articular Myofascial Release Techniques: tarsal joints, metatarsal joints, tarsal metatarsal joints, metatarsal phalangeal joints, interphalangeal joints (all toes)
5. Retinaculum Technique: tarsal tunnel
   - The technique from Step 6 is referenced as capsule, ligament, tendon, and retinaculum techniques and be can found on page 103 of this text.

Respiratory System

1. The Spinal Protocol (Steps 1 to 14.)
2. Cervical Syndrome and Neck Pain protocol (Steps 1 to 3.)
3. Shoulder Joint protocol (Steps 1 to 5.)
4. Articular Myofascial Release Technique: chest technique
5. Soft Tissue Myofascial Release Techniques: anterior/posterior holds
   - Perform wherever signs are positive for postural asymmetry, limited joint mobility (sternochondral, costochondral, costovertebral, intercostal joint), soft tissue loss of flexibility (intercostal muscles, pleura, viscera), limited ranges of motion (rib cage motion amplitude on all planes).
6. Articular Fascial Release: Rib Technique
   - Assess pump handle and bucket handle rib excursion. Perform technique wherever rib excursion is compromised.
7. Transverse Myofascial Releases: diaphragms (pelvic, Respiratory abdominal, thoracic inlet) and cranio-cervical junction
   - Techniques that are part of the Spinal Protocol are repeated here.

Shin Splints

1. The Spinal Protocol (Steps 1 to 14.)
2. Soft Tissue Myofascial Release Technique: all joints and soft tissues of the extremity involved including ankle joints and foot, proximal to distal
3. Periosteal Release: anterolateral tibia
4. Hanging Technique: tibiofibular joint
5. Articular Myofascial Release Technique: ankle joints (tibiotalar and subtalar)

Shoulder Joint Dysfunction

1. The Spinal Protocol (Steps 1 to 14.) should be considered.
   - All shoulder joint pain and disability is in some manner associated with spinal dysfunction.
2. Cervical Syndrome and Neck Pain protocol (Steps 1 to 3.)
   - All shoulder girdle problems require these steps. There is always a cervical component of dysfunction contributing in some degree to shoulder problems.
3. Soft Tissue Myofascial Release Technique: clavipectoral hold
4. Articular Myofascial Release Technique: glenohumeral joint
5. Assess mobility of scapulothoracic joint. Consider applying Articular Myofascial Release Technique at the scapulothoracic joint.

Spasticity: Synergetic Pattern Release of the Lower Quadrant

1. The Spinal Protocol (Steps 1 to 14.)
   - Pelvic balance and trunk elongation will be addressed.

2. Soft Tissue Myofascial Release Technique: The Lateral Hold: quadratus lumborum
   - This addresses the elevated pelvic component of the synergic pattern.

3. Soft Tissue Myofascial Release Technique: hip joint
   - This will addresses the hip flexion component of the synergic pattern.

4. Soft Tissue Myofascial Release Technique: medial/lateral hold of the upper thigh
   - This will addresses the adduction and internal rotation component of the synergic pattern.

5. Soft Tissue Myofascial Release Technique: knee joint
   - This addresses the knee flexion or extension component of the synergic pattern.

6. Soft Tissue Myofascial Release Technique: anterior/posterior hold of the gastrocnemius muscle belly
   - This addresses the prolonged and premature firing of the gastrocnemius contributing to the equinus foot posture.

7. Soft Tissue Myofascial Release Technique: medial/lateral hold of the tibialis anterior
   - When there is an equinovarus foot posture, there is premature and prolonged firing of the tibialis anterior.

8. Soft Tissue Myofascial Release Technique: anterior/posterior and medial/lateral holds of the ankle joint

9. Soft Tissue Myofascial Release Technique: foot and toes

10. Articular Myofascial Release Technique: hip joint

11. Articular Myofascial Release Technique: tibiofemoral joint (knee)

12. Articular Myofascial Release Technique: ankle joints (tibiotalar and subtalar)
    - Dorsiflexion must be attained. Heel loading is essential to decrease synergic pattern. When heel strike is not present, forefoot strike will occur and predispose towards clonus, extensor hypertonicty, and other typical lower quadrant synergic pattern responses.

13. Hanging Technique: tibiofibular joint

14. Articular Fascial Release Technique: all tarsal, metatarsal, tarsal metatarsal, metatarsal phalangeal and interphalangeal joints of foot and toes.

15. Patella Technique

16. Muscle Belly Technique: quadriceps, hamstring, gastrocnemius, tibialis anterior

17. ligament, capsule, tendon and retinaculum techniques as indicated
    - Strain and Counterstrain Technique as indicated. More chronic and severe spastic legs will require 2 or 3 repetitions of this protocol.

Spasticity: Synergetic Pattern Release of the Upper Quadrant

1. The Spinal Protocol (Steps 1 to 14.)

2. Cervical Syndrome and Neck Pain protocol (Steps 1 to 3.)
   - This addresses the neck flexion and side bending component of the synergic pattern.

3. Respiratory System protocol (Steps 1 to 7.)
   - This addresses the elevated and protracted shoulder girdle component of the synergic pattern.

4. Shoulder Joint Dysfunction protocol (Steps 1 to 5)
   - This addresses the shoulder flexion, adduction, and internal rotation component of the synergic pattern.

5. The Latissimum Dorsi Muscle Belly Technique (See page 101.)
   - The subluxed hemiplegic shoulder is the result of caudal depression of the humeral head by a latissimus dorsi, which is hypertonic, pulling on the humeral head within a flaccid shoulder girdle.

6. Soft Tissue Myofascial Release Technique: anterior/posterior hold of the biceps/triceps
   - This addresses the elbow flexion and shoulder flexion component of the synergic pattern.

7. Soft Tissue Myofascial Release Technique: elbow joint
   - This addresses the elbow flexion component of the synergic pattern.

8. Soft Tissue Myofascial Release Technique: forearm
   - This addresses the pronation component of the synergic pattern.

9. Soft Tissue Myofascial Release Technique: anterior/posterior hold of the wrist joint
   - This addresses the wrist flexion component of the synergic pattern.

10. Soft Tissue Myofascial Release Technique: medial/lateral hold of the wrist joint
    - This addresses the ulnar deviation component of the synergic pattern.

11. Soft Tissue Myofascial Release Technique: thenar eminence and first carpalmetacarpal joint
    - This addresses the thumb flexion and adduction component of the synergic pattern.

12. Soft Tissue Myofascial Release Technique: hand

13. Soft Tissue Myofascial Release Technique: metacarpal phalangeal joint, fingers, thumb
    - This will address the flexed fingers component of the synergic pattern.

14. Articular Myofascial Release Technique: elbow joints (humeroradial joint and humeroulnar joint)

15. Articular Myofascial Release Technique: wrist joints (radiocarpal joints, ulnar carpal joints, proximal carpal row to distal carpal row, distal carpal row to metacarpal Heads)

16. Hanging Technique: Radioulnar joint

17. Articular Myofascial Release Technique: all metacarpal joints, metacarpal phalangeal joints, interphalangeal joints

18. Muscle Belly Technique: biceps, triceps, brachioradialis, thenar eminence, hypothenar eminence

19. Capsule, ligament and retinaculum techniques as indicated

The Spinal Protocol

For low back pain, and spinal pain and disability

Low back pain is the most common orthopedic problem in North America. A multisystems approach to its treatment can be effective and efficient, so that all aspects of these complex systems can be encompassed. If low back pain is treated with Myofascial Release 3-Planer Fascial Fulcrum Approach, the following protocol can be followed. A comprehensive assessment should precede this program.

Low back pain is a joint and soft tissue problem that can affect all populations. The following protocol can be used to treat the pelvis, sacrum, and spinal joints. It includes a defacilitation of spinal cord hyperactivity. It normalizes tensions of the dura mater, mobilizes nerve roots of the spinal cord, and corrects sacral plexus impingements. When appropriate, it can be follow by other protocols.

TREATMENT

1. Articular Fascial Release Techniques: anterior and posterior iliosacral joint

   - In chronic cases, perform each technique (for anterior and posterior) twice.
   - In cases of abdominal, groin, and genital pain, perform the *anterior* release 5 times.
   - If there is bladder incontinence, perform the *anterior* release technique 4 times.
   - When there is buttock pain, perform the *posterior* 3 times.
   - If there is radicular (leg) pain, unilateral or bilateral, repeat the *posterior* release 5 times.

2. Articular Myofascial Release Technique: the sacrum

   - This technique is best applied after

Muscle Energy Technique and "Beyond" for the sacrum. (See *Integrative Manual Therapy,* Vol. III.) If biomechanical dysfunction is not addressed in this manner, repeat the Articular Myofascial Release for the sacrum 5 times.

   - For a neurologic patient (cerebral palsy, traumatic brain injury, hemiplegia, etc.), repeat this technique after every several hours of therapy. There is a fascial unwinding of the dura mater that occurs as a result of this technique, with an apparent fibrolytic effect on the brain and spinal cord tissue environment.

3. Articular Myofascial Release: the lumbo-sacral junction

   - This technique is essential for restoration of intradiscal space.
   - Reciprocal movement can be restored with this technique.
   - All clients require 4 repetitions of this technique.

4. Soft Tissue Myofascial Release Technique: the thoracolumbar junction

5. Articular Myofascial Release Technique: the thoracolumbar junction

   - Assess thoracolumbar mobility before and after applying this technique.
   - The more chronic cases may require 2 repetitions of Steps 4 and 5.
   - If the client has any respiratory, cardiac, or cardiopulmonary problems, repeat Steps 4 and 5, 3 times each.

6. Soft Tissue Myofascial Release Technique: the cervico-thoracic junction

   - When the patient has a history of cardiac, respiratory, or cardiopulmonary problems, repeat this techniques 3 times.
   - Always perform this technique before any cranial therapy is performed.

- When there are swallowing problems (dysphasia), headaches, migraines, temporomandibular problems, repeat this technique 3 times.

7. Defacilitation of the spine

   - The first time this technique is performed the purpose is to deactivate the spinal cord. This may take up to 30 or 45 minutes.

   - After the first time, this technique will only take 5 minutes or less to perform.

   - It can be used as a balancing technique for every client, within any protocol, after every several hours of therapy.

8. L5/S1 (Lumbosacral) decompression

9. Mobilization of external nerve root impingements from L5/S1

10. Cranio-cervical junction release

    - This technique is very important. It cannot be successfully completed unless Steps 2, 3, 4, 5, 6, and 7 are performed. The lumbosacral junction must be mobilized for complete mobilization of the cranio-cervical junction (occipitoatlantal joints and the suboccipital space).

    - When the patient has neurologic findings, this technique should be performed 5 times.

    - If there is any indication of cranial nerve compression, this technique should be performed 10 times (especially in case of torticollis, cranial nerve XI compression, colic and projectile vomiting, tongue thrust, lip, and other oral motor problems, cranial nerve IX and XII compression).

11. Mobilization of external nerve root impingements (e.g. cervical syndrome, sciatica)

    - This technique needs to be performed as a total spinal and dura mater release.

- If all spinal nerve root impingements have not been eradicated completely, there is no free mobility of the spinal column.

- All sacral plexus nerve roots can be mobilized with this technique.

- Filum terminale tension where it inserts on the coccyx (tethered spinal cord) can also be mobilized.

- Dural hypertrophy at the S2 insertion is also addressed with this technique. Many nerve roots may be impinged.

- This technique may require from 1 to 10 hours total duration in order to completely mobilize all nerve roots. Alternate this technique with

12. Temporomandibular joint compression and decompression

    - This technique can be alternately performed with Step 11.

    - Fascial unwinding of the dural sheaths of the nerve roots occurs with this technique.

    - Up to 5 hours total duration of this technique may be required for multiple nerve root impingements.

    - Step 11 alternated with Step 12 may totally eliminate all radicular pain of upper and lower extremities.

13. Balancing the cranial dura: lateral vault and fronto-occipital hold

    - In order to prevent headaches after fascial mobilization of the pelvis, sacrum, and spinal column, this technique must be performed.

    - This technique may be repeated whenever there is a history of headaches, migraines, facial, and temporomandibular joint pain. It is an excellent balancing technique.

14. Transverse Myofascial Release: diaphragms: pelvic, respiratory, abdominal, and thoracic inlet

   ▪ This 3-part process is an excellent balancing technique.

Total Hip Replacement

(Acute, In-Hospital, Initial Day After Surgery)

TREATMENT

1. The Spinal Protocol (Steps 1 to 14.)

2. Soft Tissue Myofascial Release Technique: knee joint on the side that has been operated upon

3. Articular Fascial Release Technique: knee joint on the side that has been operated upon

4. Soft Tissue Myofascial Release Technique: ankle and foot on the side that has been operated upon

5. Articular Myofascial Release Technique: ankle joints (tibiotalar and subtalar) foot joints on the side that has been operated upon

   ▪ Dorsiflexion must be attained to at least 10 degrees

6. Soft Tissue Myofascial Release Technique: hip joint that has been operated upon

7. Muscle Belly Technique: hamstrings, quadriceps, gastrocnemius, tibialis anterior on the side that has been operated upon

Total Knee Replacement

(Acute, In-hospital, Initial Day After Surgery)

TREATMENT

1. The Spinal Protocol (Steps 1 to 14.)
2. Soft Tissue Myofascial Release Technique: hip joint on the side that has been operated upon
3. Articular Myofascial Release Technique: hip joint on the side that has been operated upon
4. Soft Tissue Myofascial Release Technique: ankle and foot on the side that has been operated upon
5. Articular Fascial Release Technique: tibiotalar and subtalar foot joints (ankle joints) on the side that has been operated upon
   - Dorsiflexion must be obtained to at least up to 10 degrees.
6. Soft Tissue Myofascial Release Technique: knee joint, the joint that has been operated upon
7. Muscle Belly Technique: hamstrings, quadriceps, gastrocnemius, tibialis anterior, peroneals, on the side that has been operated upon

The Treatment of a Patient with Low Back Pain Using an Integrated Systems Approach

A male client arrives for evaluation and treatment. His complaints include: ten years of low back pain,with intermittent left leg pain during the three years prior to evaluation. He has a history of headaches since childhood, but they have been contained with medication. He has suffered from indigestion with heartburn and some stomach cramps for one year, and he is concerned that the stress of his job will continue to cause this indigestion. He is thirty-five years old. He plays racquetball once a week. He stopped smoking six years ago. He sleeps well. His family is important to him. He goes to his children's sports and education events. He likes to ski and does not vacation enough.

Initially, the therapist finds mild postural asymmetry, low back and cervical movement dysfunction, mild weakness of the left foot and lower extremity musculature, and limited left leg range of motion. Biomechanics are addressed. Muscle Energy and 'Beyond' Technique is performed. Pelvic dysfunction (a left upslip and a right outflare) is corrected. Sacral dysfunction is addressed. A left descended sacrum, a left posterior vertical rotation of the sacrum, bilateral extended sacrum, unilateral flexed sacrum on the right, and a left on right sacral torsion are corrected. Some flexed and extended Type I dysfunction is addressed. Occipitoatlantal and atlantoaxial joint dysfunction are corrected. Postural symmetry is restored. Lower extremity pain is eliminated. Range of spinal motion is increased almost to normal. Back pain decreases by 30 percent. This occurs during 4 hours of treatment. (4 sessions of 1 hour each.)

Strain and Counterstrain is then performed to eliminate protective muscle spasm. The hypertonicity of the following muscles is addressed: bilateral iliacus, bilateral hamstring, bilateral gastrocnemius, anterior L5, anterior T12 left, anterior T4, elevated left first rib, O/M left. After one hour of treatment, lower extremity ranges of motion are within normal limits and pain-free. Spinal extension (cervical, thoracic, lumbar and lumbosacral) is almost pain-free in outer ranges. Back pain is reduced by 70 percent.

The Spinal Protocol is now performed once (Steps 1 to 14.). After 4 hours (4 sessions of 1 hour each), Myofascial Release is complete, the patient is totally pain free without any heartburn or indigestion. He stops using his headache medications. He describes less stress, improved productivity at work, and less tension at home.

Advanced Strain and Counterstrain Technique is performed during one treatment session. The client responds well to the following techniques: Aorta, Vena Cava, Iliac Arteries bilateral, and Femoral Arteries bilateral. He immediately reports increased energy, an ability to stand straighter with decreased tension in both legs.

Cranial Therapy is performed during one treatment session. Visceral Manipulation is then performed during a 30 minute session, focusing on tensions around the medial pericardial ligaments, the cardiac sphincter, and the hepatogastric ligaments of the lesser omentum.

The patient is discharged pain-free and fully functional, with exceptional client satisfaction. After 6 months he is still pain-free, medication-free, and fully functional.

PART SIX

RESEARCH

CHAPTER 26

INCREASING RANGE OF MOTION WITH MYOFASCIAL RELEASE

The following research are excerpts from *Developmental Manual Therapy for Physical Rehabilitation for the Neurologic Patient*, Vol. I, II, Weiselfish, Sharon Honey. Ph.D., The Union Institute, 1992, copyright 1993 by Weiselfish, Sharon Honey, Ph.D., UMI Dissertation Series, Ann Arbor, Michigan, modified for this volume.

A Statistical Analysis of a Quantitative Research Study With Neurologic Clients as Subjects

Developmental Manual Therapy

Utilization of Manual and CranioSacral Therapy for treatment of the neurologic patient, results in a process of normalization. The amount of progress and the speed of progress appear dependent on the severity and the chronicity of the neuromusculoskeletal dysfunction. Without the intervention of Integrative Manual Therapy, the anticipated process of recovery for a patient suffering from a traumatic brain injury appears to follow the *Glasgow Coma Scale/Ranchos Los Amigos Scale*. When Integrative Manual Therapy is implemented to provide Structural Rehabilitation with an Integrated Systems Approach for correction of neuromusculoskeletal dysfunction, the patient's process of recovery does not always adhere to the criteria of the *Glasgow Coma Scale/Ranchos Los Amigos Scale*.

The effectiveness of Integrative Manual Therapy is a function of the skill of the practitioner. The accuracy of the differential diagnosis of primary dysfunctions also is greater with the greater expertise of the practitioner. With increased expertise and practice, the practitioner develops the knowledge and skill to treat the primary areas of dysfunction first, whether those dysfunctions are biomechanical, muscular, fascial, neural or vas-

cular. When primary dysfunctions are treated first, results are more effective and efficient.

Recovery with Integrative Manual Therapy is a process of normalization. Body systems normalize; body functions normalize. This process of normalization continues as long as the practitioner, or the combination of practitioners and health care professionals can provide all the intervention needed to address all the dysfunction in all body systems. Depending on the sites of the injuries and which unique primary dysfunction the patient presents with (these are always unique to each patient), the patient will recover function according to function lost. Occasionally motor function will begin to normalize first; occasionally cognitive function will recover first. This is ultimately dependent on the severity, number, and sites of injuries.

As the patient receives treatment with Structural Rehabilitation, the healing of the neuromusculoskeletal systems continues and the potential for function increases. If the Functional Rehabilitation process is also dysfunction, and function-specific with a focus on functional outcomes, the patient will fulfill his or her new potential and will continually and consistently make gains.

For patients with more chronic and severe problems, there does not appear to be a plateau with Integrative Manual Therapy where improvement ceases. These patients continue to show improvement—occasionally small gains, occasionally quantum leaps in progress—but they never cease to present progress in at least some minor functional capacity.

This process of normalization is uniquely induced by rehabilitation intervention which provides Structural *and* Functional therapy. The results of rehabilitation are consistent for the early, post-acute patient (less than two years status post neurologic insult) and for the late post-acute patient (more than two years status post neurologic insult). Habilitation programs for the neuropediatric client present similar results of normalization.

The following study portrays this process of normalization of joint mobility utilizing Myofascial Release, a 3-Planar Fascial Fulcrum Approach. The outcomes of this study illustrate the potential recovery process for a neurologic patient.

A 3-Planar Fascial Fulcrum Approach to Facilitate a Process of Normalization for the Chronic Neurologic Patient

In this study, the physical therapist measures ranges of motions to document changes in a patient's mobility as one objective measure of improvement or regression in motor status. The approach assumes that measured increases in degrees of joint mobility reflect an improvement in the patient's musculoskeletal status. The purpose of this study is threefold: First, it examines the effects of Myofascial Release: A 3-Planar Fascial Fulcrum Approach on join mobility. Second, it documents ranges of motion for the neurologic patient as a normalization process. Third, it is argued that a technique which can affect the range of motion of more extensive body areas, influencing more tissues and structures than the localized areas being treated, might be more cost effective for institutions to implement.

(Key words: Neurologic patient, Range of motion, Soft Tissue Myofascial Release, Articular Myofascial Release, Normalization process, Fulcrum.)

A rehabilitation assessment of the *neurologic* patient typically observes motor behavior, including passive and active range of motion. Techniques to improve and occasionally to maintain joint mobility are commonly integrated into the therapeutic program. Physical therapists assign exercises to maintain and increase passive range of motion. These exercises affect the intra-articular and extra-articular tissues (capsules, ligaments, tendons) as well as the soft tissue (muscle and connective tissue) of the treated body part. Therapists also commonly apply joint mobilization techniques. Mobilization affects intra-articular and extra-articular tissues. Joint mobilizations have a more limited affect on the muscle and fascia of the total body.

Since Myofascial Release is a manual therapy approach designed to affect the continuous, contiguous system of connective tissue that envelops every cell and fiber in the body, it can be utilized to increase passive range of motion. Because of the continuity of connective tissue system, the effects of tissue tension release may not be limited to the joint or the treated body part.

In this study, ten neurologic patients, all with severe, post-acute traumatic brain injuries (more than two years status posttraumatic brain injury) were treated with Myofascial Release. The treated body regions were measured for changes in ranges of motion resulting from the manual therapy. The untreated body areas were also tested for changes in ranges of motion in order to observe if this technique affected more of the total body than the specific areas treated.

Neurologic patients commonly present a synergic pattern of spasticity that inhibits movement and contributes to decreased joint mobility and ranges of motion. Physical therapists treating a neurologic patient, utilizing passive range of motion of joint mobilization exercises, observe whether the therapeutic results of Myofascial Release are also limited to the treated joints. An approach that provides beneficial effects on multiple body parts might be more cost effective than more traditional approaches such as range of motion and joint mobilization.

Ranges of motion are typically measured with a goniometer. Therapists document any increase or decrease in degrees of mobility as indicated by goniometric measurements. The success of a therapeutic intervention is typically measured by the increase in degrees of mobility attained with the therapy as measured by the goniometer. This measurement and interpretation process is generally an accepted standard for all patient populations: orthopedic, pediatric, neurologic, and others.

Pathological Neutral as an Indicator

Neurologic patients with typical synergic patterns of spasticity exhibit typical patterns of limitation in range of motion. Certain joints commonly present with a typical gross limitation of motion in one specific direction. For example, compare a healthy wrist joint with a dysfunctional wrist joint. The comparison is different from a comparison between a healthy wrist joint and the spastic wrist joint of a neurologic patient.

This joint might present with a gross postural deviation, even a deformity. The typical gross deviation patterns show excessive mobility in specific directions. These patterns are commonly present in patients with severe neurologic findings, in the following joint movement directions:

1. Shoulder adduction
2. Elbow flexion
3. Wrist flexion
4. Hip adduction
5. Ankle plantar flexion
6. Ankle inversion

Hip internal rotation and forearm pronation are often in similar distorted patterns. Patients can exhibit knee flexion synergy or extension

Table IV

Wrist Joint Range of Motion: Normal, Dysfunctional, Spastic

Healthy Wrist Joint

Plane of motion: Sagittal plane: Extension ⟷ Flexion

70°	60°	50°	40°	30°	20°	10°	0°	10°	20°	30°	40°	50°	60°	70°	80°
|							|								|
Extension 100%*							Normal Neutral								Flexion 100%*

Dysfunctional Wrist Joint

Plane of Motion: Extension ⟷ Flexion: Limitations in both direction of the sagittal plane. The pathologic neutral is displaced from neutral.

70°	60°	50°	40°	30°	20°	10°	0°	10°	20°	30°	40°	50°	60°	70°	80°
|				|			|		|					|	|
Extension 100%*							Normal Neutral								Flexion 100%*
				Barrier in Extension					Pathologic Neutral in Flexion					Barrier in Flexion	

Spastic Wrist Joint of a Neurologic Patient

Plane of motion: Extension ⟷ Flexion: Gross limitations of motion in only one direction of movement on the sagittal plane. Range of motion in the opposite direction is often excessive. The pathological neutral is grossly distant from normal.

70°	60°	50°	40°	30°	20°	10°	0°	10°	20°	30°	40°	50°	60°	70°	80°
|							|				|		|		|
Extension 100%*							Normal Neutral								Flexion 100%*
											Barrier in Flexion		Pathologic Neutral in Flexion		

* within normal limits

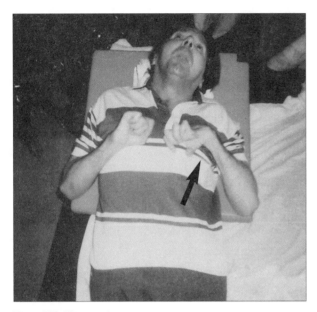

Figure 132. Wrist extension synergy.

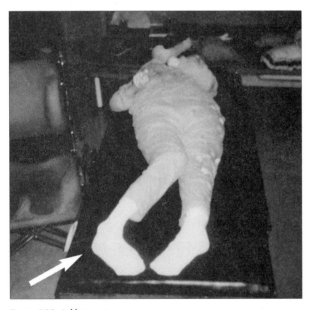

Figure 133. Ankle inversion pattern.

synergy, and occasionally wrist extension synergy, which are also commonly found in the pattern of hypomobility. See Figure 132 for wrist flexion patterns; see Figure 133 for ankle inversion pattern.

Normalization of Motion

In the case of the wrist flexion patterns, a treatment technique which results in decreased left wrist flexion would promote the normalization of wrist joint mobility, especially if the negative change in degrees of mobility occurs concurrently with an increase in degrees of mobility of left wrist extension.

In the case of ankle inversion patterns, a treatment technique that results in decreased degrees of right ankle inversion would be therapeutically beneficial, especially if concurrent with an increase in degrees of ankle eversion. This would be therapeutically more effective than an overall increase in degrees of mobility in all directions on all planes.

A purpose of this study was to present and observe Myofascial Release as a process of normalization of range of motion for the neurologic patient. Normalization would result in decreased postural deviations and deformities. A less severe pathologic neutral on one or more planes of motion needs to occur. In the case of wrist flexion patterns, this would mean an increase in left wrist extension with a decrease in left wrist flexion. In the case of ankle inversion patterns, this would mean a decrease in the equinovarus posture: decreased plantar flexion and decreased inversion.

Procedure

Myofascial Release: A 3-Planar Fascial Fulcrum Approach was utilized. Two specific techniques were performed: Soft Tissue Myofascial Release and Articular Myofascial Release technique.

This Fascial Fulcrum Technique is a 3-Planar process, performed at areas of decreased soft tissue and joint mobility. The technique is as follows:

The Soft Tissue Myofascial Release Technique: A 3-Planar Concept

POSITION

- Hands are positioned in a "sandwich" formation, on both sides of the body part to be treated (anterior/posterior or medial/lateral).

TREATMENT

1. The body part is compressed with minimal force (5 grams of force; not enough force to burst a soap bubble).

2. The hands are moved in opposite directions in order to distort the body tissue between the hands. This distortion of the body tissues occurs on three planes, one plane at a time. The hands do not move on the skin. Distortion of the internal tissues is the objective.

3. The hands displace the tissue in an indirect manner in the direction of ease, i.e., the direction of greatest tissue mobility, greatest tissue flexibility, least restriction, and least inhibition.

4. The planes of distortion are "stacked," one plane at a time until the "fulcrum" is attained.

5. *The Fulcrum:* This is the fixed point around which the tissue unwinds. The minimal compression forces are maintained. The forces, which displaced the position of the tissue on three planes, are maintained. The culmination of these forces is the fulcrum around which the fascial tissue will unwind.

6. *The Release:* The fulcrum is maintained throughout the technique. The hands do not move as the tissue movement occurs (although the temptation to move the hands is often great). The goal is *not* a physiologic unwinding of a body part. The objective is the internal "unraveling" of the fascial tissue. By maintaining the fulcrum, the force of energy contributing to the fascial release will produce more effective and efficient changes in the internal environment, i.e., the connective tissue.

The internal fascial unwinding is slow and gentle. Quick, repetitive, and forceful physiologic movements are not allowed. If the patient begins to move any body part quickly, with repetition, or with force, the practitioner asks the patient not to move. The body parts are allowed to slowly and gently change position in space. At the end of the release the hands will be in different positions because of the unwinding of the body tissues within. The body parts will be in a more normal anatomical neutral.

(For further explanation of this technique, refer to the example in the following section).

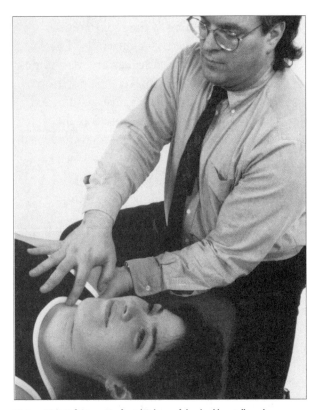

Figure 134. Soft Tissue Myofascial Release of the shoulder girdle and clavipectoral fascia.

Example:
Soft Tissue Myofascial Release of the Clavipectoral Fascia of the Shoulder Girdle

INDICATION

Protracted shoulder girdle posture and limitation in shoulder girdle and shoulder joint ranges of motion.

POSITION

- Supine or sitting.
- One hand of the therapist is posterior to scapula. The fingers are spread apart contacting as much tissue as possible. The heel of the hand (thenar and hypothenar eminences) contacts the humeral head. The other hand of the therapist rests on the clavipectoral region of that side. The same fingers can contact supraclavicular tissue, clavicle, and infraclavicular tissue and ribs.

TREATMENT

1. Compression of the clavipectoral region with both hands squeezing gently, imaging a soap bubble between the hands. This gentle compression is maintained throughout the technique.

2. *First Plane:* The anterior hand mobilizes the tissue in a cephalad direction while the posterior hand moves the tissue in a caudad direction (causing a distortion of the soap bubble). The hands return to neutral and reverse directions: the anterior hand moves the tissues in a caudad direction while the posterior hand moves the tissues in a cephalad direction. The directions (cephalad/caudad or caudad/cephalad) of the greatest mobility with the least restrictions are determined. The hands are moved in the "indirect" direction of ease. The hands maintain this new position.

3. *Second Plane:* The second plane movements are not "stacked." The hands and the tissues are not returned to neutral. The first plane tissue distortion pattern is maintained. The tissue is now moved with the anterior hand in a medial direction while the posterior hand moves the tissue in a lateral direction. The hands return to neutral on this plane and compare the ease of tissue mobility to when the anterior hand moves the tissue in a lateral direction while the posterior hands move the tissues in a medial direction. The directions (medial/lateral or lateral/medial) of the greatest mobility and least restrictions are determined. The tissue is retuned to that position.

4. *Third Plane:* The third plane motions are now "stacked." The hands and the tissues are not returned to neutral. The first and second plane tissue distortions are maintained. The tissue is now moved in a clockwise direction with the anterior hand while the posterior hand moves the tissue in a counterclockwise direction. The tissue is then returned to neutral on this plane; the opposite tissue distortion pattern is compared. The tissue is now moved in a counterclockwise direction with the anterior hand while the posterior hand moves the tissue in a clockwise direction. The two different tissue distortion patterns (clockwise/counterclockwise and counterclockwise/clockwise) are compared. The indirect pattern of tissue distortion is determined. The tissues are moved into the direction of distortion.

5. *The Fulcrum:* Up to this point, each hand has exerted four different mechanical forces on the body to distort the tissue between then hands. The directions of force are:

- Compression
- Superior or inferior
- Medial or lateral
- Clockwise or counterclockwise (medial rotation/lateral rotation).

Each hand now maintains all four directions of force, also maintaining a fulcrum for the tissue unwinding, for the duration of the application of the technique.

6. *The Release:* Maintain the fulcrum. As the tissue unwinds and movement occurs in the body's internal environment, there is a temptation to move the hands and release the fulcrum. *The temptation must be resisted.* The therapist and patient may perceive heat, paresthesia, anesthesia, vibration, fatigue, electricity, cold, perspiration, pain, circulatory changes, breathing changes, sympathetic skin erythremia or blanching, and other phenomena. Do not release the fulcrum. By the end of the application of the technique the signs and symptoms will subside. When all movement, signs, symptoms, and perceptions have ceased, the technique is complete.

RESULT

Increased range of motion.

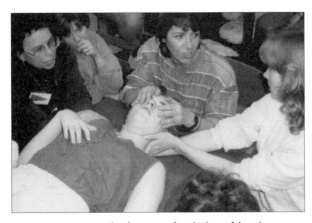

Figure 135. Treatment with Soft Tissue Myofascial Release of the right glenohumeral joint.

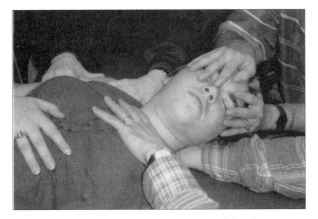

Figure 136. Treatment with Articular Myofascial Release of the right glenohumeral joint.

Example:
Articular Myofascial Release of the Glenohumeral Joint

INDICATION

Limitations of glenohumeral joint movements.

POSITION

- Supine or sitting.
- One hand of the therapist grips the shoulder girdle to control the position of the glenoid fossa. The other hand grips the upper arm to control the position of the humeral head. Joint surfaces are not distracted or approximated.

TREATMENT

1. *First Plane:* The superior hand on the shoulder girdle pulls the glenoid fossa cephalad while the inferior hand on the upper arm pulls the humeral head caudad. The articular surfaces are then returned to neutral. Now the directions are reversed: the superior hand pushes the glenoid fossa caudad while the inferior hand pushes the humeral head cephalad. A comparison is made: Which pattern of directions (cephalad/caudad or caudad/cephalad) was the most mobile? The joint surfaces are returned to the positions of greater mobility. The positions of the articular surfaces on the plane are maintained.

2. *Second Plane:* The second plane movements are "stacked." The superior hand holding the shoulder girdle can push the glenoid fossa in an anterior direction while the inferior hand holding the upper arm can push the humeral head in a posterior direction. The articular surfaces are then returned to neutral. Now the directions of displacement of the articular surfaces are reversed: the superior hand pushes the

glenoid fossa in a posterior direction while the inferior hand pushes the humeral head in an anterior direction. The displacement patterns (anterior/posterior or posterior/ anterior) are compared. The joint surfaces are moved in the indirect directions of ease. The articular surfaces are maintained in this new position.

3. *Third Plane:* The third plane movements are "stacked." The superior hand gripping the shoulder girdle rotates the glenoid fossa in an external direction of rotation while the inferior hand gripping the upper arm rotates the humeral head in an internal direction. The articular surfaces are then returned to neutral and the directions of displacement are reversed: the superior hand pushes the glenoid fossa into an internal direction of rotation while the inferior hand moves the humeral head into external rotation. The patterns of displacement (external/internal rotations or internal/external rotations) are compared. The articular surfaces on this plane are moved in the direction of greatest mobility, least resistance. The positions of the articular surfaces on the plane are maintained.

4. *The Fulcrum:* Each hand mechanically exerts three different directions of forces to position the articular surfaces in opposite directions on three planes. Each hand maintains all three directions of forces, maintaining a fulcrum for the tissue unwinding of the joint capsule and ligaments throughout the duration of the technique.

5. *The Release:* Maintain the fulcrum. As the tissue unwinds and sensations of extra-articular and intra-articular movement are perceived, there is a temptation to move the hands and release the fulcrum. *This temptation to release the fulcrum must be resisted.* The fulcrum is maintained until all movements, all signs, all symptoms, and all perceptions have ceased.

RESULT

Improved articular balance. Neutral balance of the humeral head within the glenoid fossa will be more normal; joint mobility will be increased; range of shoulder motions will be increased.

Table VI

Number of Treated and Untreated Joints Measured in Ten Treated Patients

	Treated Joints			Untreated Joints		
	Left	Right	Total	Left	Right	Total
Hip	5	4	9	5	6	11
Knee	5	3	8	5	7	12
Ankle	6	5	11	4	4	8
Shoulder	4	3	7	5	7	12
Elbow	1	0	1	9	10	19
Wrist	3	2	5	7	7	14
TOTAL	24	7	4	35	4	76
	58.5%	41.5%	100%	46%	53.9%	100%

Method

Ten subjects with severe late post-acute traumatic brain injury, who were inpatients at a long-term care facility, participated in this study. Participants included four women and six men. Years of injuries were: 1968, 1979, 1983, 1986, 1987, 1988, and 1989.

Joints treated with Myofascial Release included: hip joints, knee joints, ankle joints, shoulder joints, elbow joints, and wrist joints. Twenty-four left side joints were treated (58.5 percent) and 17 right side joint were treated (41.5 percent). Forty-one treated joints were measured before and after treatment by impartial therapists. The practitioners also measured the untreated joints (before and after Myofascial Release techniques were performed on the 41 treated joints). Thirty-five left-side, untreated joints were measured (46.1 percent). Forty-one right-side untreated joint were measured (53.9 percent). (See Table VI.)

Directions of motion were measured at the treated and untreated joints before and after Myofascial Release techniques were performed. Six directions of movement on three planes were measured at the treated and untreated hip joints:

flexion, extension, adduction, abduction, internal rotation, and external rotation. Two directions of movement on one plane were measured at the knee joints: flexion and extension. Four directions of movement on two planes were measured at the ankle joints: planar flexion, dorsiflexion, inversion and eversion. Six directions of movement on the three planes were measured at the shoulder joints: flexion, extension, adduction, abduction, internal rotation and external rotation. Two directions of movement on one plane were measured at the elbow joints: flexion and extension. Two directions of movement were measured on one plane at the wrist joints: flexion and extension.

At the treated joints, 83 (55.7 percent) directions of movement were measured on the left side, and 66 (44.3 percent) directions of movement were measure on the right side. At the untreated joints, 108 (45.4 percent directions of movement were measured on the left side, and 130 (54.6 percent) directions of movement were measured on the right side. Multiple directions of movement were measured in order to observe the more far-reaching *effects* of the 3-Planar Myofascial Fulcrum Techniques. (See Table VII.)

Table VII

Number of Movements Measured in Treated and Untreated Joints in Ten Treated Patients

	Treated Joints		Untreated Joints	
	Left	Right	Left	Right
Hip flexion	5	4	5	5
Hip extension	2	2	4	5
Hip adduction	4	3	5	5
Hip abduction	4	4	5	5
Hip internal rotation	4	4	5	5
Hip external rotation	4	4	5	5
Knee extension	4	3	5	7
Knee Flexion	5	3	5	6
Ankle Plantar flexion	6	5	4	4
Ankle dorsiflexion	5	5	2	4
Ankle inversion	6	5	4	4
Ankle eversion	6	5	3	4
Shoulder flexion	4	3	5	7
Shoulder adduction	4	3	5	7
Shoulder abduction	4	3	5	7
Shoulder internal rotation	4	3	4	7
Shoulder external rotation	4	3	4	7
Elbow extension	1	0	9	10
Elbow flexion	1	0	9	10
Wrist extension	3	2	7	7
Wrist flexion	3	2	7	7
TOTAL	83	66	108	130
	55.7%	44.3%	45.4%	54.6%

Interpretations of the data for conclusion regarding "normalization" of ranges of motion used the following standards of normal mobility. (See Table VIII.)

Table VIII
Standards of Normal Mobility

Hip	Flexion	0–125
	Extension	0–10
	Adduction	0–30
	Abduction	0–45
	Internal Rotation	0–45
	External Rotation	0–45
Knee	Extension	0
	Flexion	0–140
Ankle	Plantar Flexion	0–45
	Dorsi Flexion	0–20
Foot	Inversion	0–40
	Eversion	0–20
Shoulder	Extension	0–45
	Flexion	0–180
	Adduction	0
	Abduction	0–180
	Internal Rotation	0–90
	External Rotation	0–90
Elbow	Extension	0
	Flexion	0–145
Wrist	Extension	0–70
	Flexion	0–80

Therapists used goniometers to measure movements before and after treatment. Changes in degrees of mobility were documented as:

- Increased degrees of joint mobility
- Decreased degrees of joint mobility
- No change in degrees of joint mobility

If measured changes of joint mobility were +2 degrees, this was documented as no change in joint mobility. All increases in degrees of mobility

were interpreted as normal, except for those directions of movements that were excessive as shown in Figures 132 and 133, where increased degrees of mobility would have resulted in increased postural deviation and deformity into the synergic pattern of spasticity. The degrees of mobility in these directions of motion are compared to the Standards of Normal Mobility presented in Table 3. The directions of movement, which required negative degrees of mobility changes for normalization included: hip adduction, hip internal rotation, knee flexion, ankle plantar flexion, ankle inversion, shoulder adduction elbow flexion, and wrist flexion.

Results

The Myofascial Release Techniques affected all patients. Of the treated joints, 96 (64 percent) of the measured directions of movement changed to more normal; 17 (11 percent) of the measured direction of movement changed to less normal; 36 (24 percent) of the measured directions of movement showed no change. (Differences of +2 degrees were documented as no change.) Of the untreated joints, 136 (57 percent) of the measured directions of movement changed to more normal, 32 (13 percent) of the measured directions of movement changed to less normal, and 71 (30 percent) of the measured direction of movement showed no change. (Differences of +2 degrees were documented as no change.) (See Table IX.)

All joints displayed increase mobility after treatment. The distribution of the *normalization process* in Treated and Untreated Joints by directions of movements measured can be seen in Table X.

Discussion

When a neurologic patient is treated with passive ranges of motion or joint mobilization techniques, the local tissues and structures directly addressed with therapy are affected. Changes in joint mobility and ranges of motion will typically be observed

Table IX

Distribution of *Normalization Process* In Treated and Untreated Joints for All Directions of Movement Measured by Joint, Number and Percent

	Treated Joints						Untreated Joints					
	Change to More Normal		Change to Less Normal		No Change (within 2°)		Change to More Normal		Change to Less Normal		No Change (within 2°)	
Hip	32	73%	3	7%	9	20%	34	58%	8	14%	17	29%
Knee	7	47%	0	0%	8	53%	13	57%	1	4%	9	39%
Ankle	27	63%	5	12%	11	26%	16	55%	3	10%	10	34%
Shoulder	21	60%	9	26%	5	14%	29	48%	11	18%	21	34%
Elbow	2	100%	0	0%	0	0%	26	68%	5	13%	7	18%
Wrist	7	70%	0	0%	3	30%	17	61%	4	14%	7	25%
TOTAL	96	64%	17	11%	36	24%	135	57%	31	13%	71	30%

specifically at the localized treated joint or joints after therapy. The techniques ordinarily applied are direct approaches: stretching/pulling/pushing against the barrier, against tissue resistance, often requiring energy exertion of the therapist, and occasionally causing discomfort for the patient.

The 3-Planar Fascial Fulcrum Approach is an indirect approach. It does not force the tissue, requires minimal energy exertion of the therapist, and causes minimal discomfort.

The results of the study indicated that Soft Tissue Myofascial Release and Articular Fascial Release are effective techniques to increase ranges of motion in the severe and chronic neurologic patient with gross postural deviation and deformities.

The study results indicate that the 3-Planar Fascial Fulcrum Approach has extensive effects and is capable of affecting ranges of motion in body parts that are not treated. This is possibly due to the anatomic continuity of the fascial tissue. This might result in less time spent by therapists in attaining and maintain ranges of motion in heath care facilities with severely impaired patients.

A process of normalization is presented for consideration. The neurologic patient population with severe spasticity is unique: increased degrees of mobility in all directions on all three planes are not always beneficial for this patient population. Often this would mean an increase in gross postural deviations and deformities. This Indirect 3-Planar Fascial Fulcrum Approach results in a normalization of tissue tension. The results of this study show an increase in degrees of mobility when appropriate and a decrease in degrees of mobility when appropriate, attained by these treatment techniques.

Because the fascial system is a total body, continuous, and contiguous system, effects on other body systems and other body functions often occur.

Table X

Distribution of *Normalization Process* In Treated and Untreated Joints by Directions of Movement Measured, Number and Percent

	Treated Joints						Untreated Joints					
	Change to More Normal		Change to Less Normal		No Change (within 2°)		Change to More Normal		Change to Less Normal		No Change (within 2°)	
Hip												
Flexion	77.8	7			22.2	2	50.1	5			50.0	5
Extension	25.0	1	75.0	3			22.5	2	33.3	3	44.4	4
Adduction	42.9	2			57.1	4	60.0	6	10.0	1	30.0	3
Abduction	75.0	6			25.0	2	40.0	4	40.0	4	20.0	2
Int'l Rotation	100.0	8					80.0	8			20.0	2
Ext'l Rotation	87.5	7			12.5	1	80.0	8			20.0	2
Knee												
Extension	14.3	1			85.7	6	41.7	5	8.3	1	50.0	6
Flexion	75.0	6			25.0	2	72.7	8			27.3	3
Ankle												
Plantar Flexion	72.7	8			27.3	3	50.0	4			50.0	4
Dorsiflexion	50.0	5	20.2	2	30.3	3	50.0	3	16.7	1	33.3	2
Inversion	90.0	10			9.1	1	62.5	5			37.5	3
Eversion	36.4	4	27.3	3	36.4	4	57.1	4	28.6	2	14.3	1
Shoulder												
Extension											100.0	3
Flexion	57.1	4	42.9	3			58.3	7	16.7	2	25.0	3
Adduction	85.7	6			14.3	1	66.7	8			33.3	4
Abduction	42.9	3	42.9	3	14.3	1	33.3	4	33.3	4	33.3	4
Int'l Rotation	85.7	6			14.3	1	54.6	6	9.1	1	36.4	4
Ext'l Rotation	28.6	2	42.9	3	28.6	2	36.4	4	36.4	4	27.3	3
Elbow												
Extension	100.0	1					52.6	10	21.1	4	26.3	5
Flexion	100.0	1					84.2	16	5.3	1	10.5	2
Wrist												
Extension	60.0	3			40.0	2	50.0	7	28.6	4	21.4	3
Flexion	80.0	4			20.0	1	71.4	10			28.6	4
Total	64.4	96	11.4	17	24.2	36	56.3	134	13.4	32	30.3	72

Table XI

Summary Statistics for Motions Which Became More Normal[1] in Treated and Untreated Patients
number of patients (N), mean + standard deviation (sd), medical range (minimum–maximum) for absolute value of difference (post–pre)[2]

Motion	Treated Joints			Untreated Joints		
	N	Mean + sd	Median, range	N	Mean + sd	Median, range
Hip						
Flexion	7	11. 6+ 6.7	10, 4–24	5	11.4 + 4.7	13, 4–16
Extension	1	6.0 + 0	6, 6–6	2	8.0 + 2.8	8, 6–10
Adduction	3	15.3 + 10.0	16, 5–25	6	6.7 + 2.7	6, 4–10
Abduction	6	6.3 + 2.4	6, 4–10	4	6.3 + 2.9	5.5, 4–10
Internal Rotation	8	11.1 + 10.1	6.5, 4–34	8	14.5 + 12.4	11, 4–40
External Rotation	7	15.4 + 7.9	16, 5–28	8	11.9 + 7.0	10, 5–26
Knee						
Extension	1	8.0 + 0	8, 8–8	5	13.0 + 15.8	5, 4–41
Flexion	6	11.3 + 8.9	9, 5–29	8	12.4 + 7.1	12.5, 3–23
Ankle						
Plantar Flexion	8	7.0 + 2.8	6, 4–12	4	10.0 + 5.7	8, 6–18
Dorsi Flexion	5	18.4 + 18.5	8, 6–50	3	7.3 + 2.3	6, 6–10
Inversion	10	14.2 + 10.3	11, 4–40	5	11.2 + +5.2	10, 6–20
Eversion	4	13.5 + 11.2	12, 4–26	4	13.5 + 5.3	15, 6–18
Shoulder						
Extension	0			0		
Flexion	4	21.3 + 14.4	17.5, 10–40	7	18.0 + 5.7	20, 10–25
Adduction	6	14.2 + 14.3	5, 5–35	8	10.3 + 9.9	6.5, 5–34
Abduction	3	15.0 + 17.3	17.5, 5–45	4	17.0 + 20.8	7.5, 5–48
Internal Rotation	6	20.8 + 13.6	7.5, 5–10	6	15.7 + 8.2	12.5, 9–30
External Rotation	2	7.5 + 3.5	10, 10–10	4	12.0 + 12.1	6.5, 5–30
Elbow						
Extension	1	10.2 + 0	5, 5–5	10	11.4 + 5.9	10, 4–20
Flexion	1	5.0 + 0	20, 15–25	16	10.3 + 7.2	7.5, 3–25
Wrist						
Extension	3	20.0 + 5.0	7.5, 5–70	7	17.0 + 8.8	20, 4–25
Flexion	4	22.5 + 31.8		10	13.1 + 6.1	12, 5–22

[1] Improvement of at least three degrees.

[2] Absolute value of improvement was used because for some motions, a negative difference meant improvement.

CHAPTER 27

A PICTORIAL CASE STUDY
TREATMENT OF A LATE POST-ACUTE PEDIATRIC PATIENT

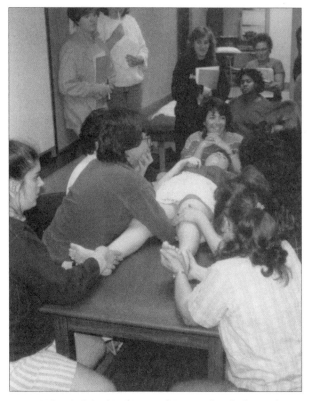

Figure 137. Multiple hands performing Soft Tissue Myofascial Release and a De-facilitation of the Spine Technique.

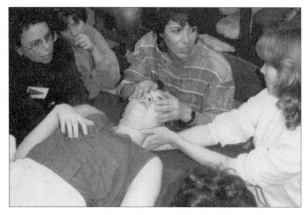

Figure 138. Myofascial Release performed at multiple regions: A. Soft Tissue Myofascial Release of the neck; B. Soft Tissue Myofascial Release of the right shoulder; C. Neurofascial Release on a Sagittal Plane.

Case Study

A Soft Tissue Myofascial Release and Articular Myofascial Release was used for treatment of a late post-acute pediatric patient. (A multiple hands treatment session was utilized.)

History

This 11-year-old girl has been receiving long-term functional rehabilitation prior to this treatment session of Structural Rehabilitation.

Goal

To improve posture, mobility, tone and function.

TREATMENT SESSION

Figure 137 shows multiple hands performing Soft TissueMyofascial Release and De-facilitation of the spine to decrease hypertonicity followed by Decompression of L5/S1.

Figure 138 shows Soft Tissue Myofascial Release of the neck; Articular Fascial Release of the right shoulder and Neurofascial Release on a sagittal plane.

Figure 139 shows Transverse Fascial Release of the Respiratory Abdominal Diaphragm, and the Thoracic Inlet with Neurofascial Release: Sagittal Plane, and Articular Fascial Release of the Right Glenohumeral Joint

Note changes in head and neck posture, left shoulder girdle protraction, right elbow and wrist flexion contracture, left thumb and fingers spasticity, right foot talar inversion, left knee and ankle articular balance.

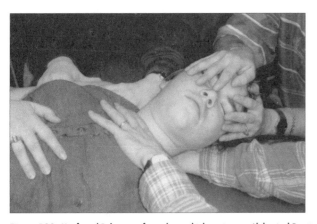

Figure 139. Myofascial Release performed at multiple regions: a. Abdominal Respiratory Diaphragm Release; b. Thoracic Inlet Diaphragm Release; c. Neurofascial Release on a Sagittal Plane; d. Articular Myofascial Release of the right shoulder.

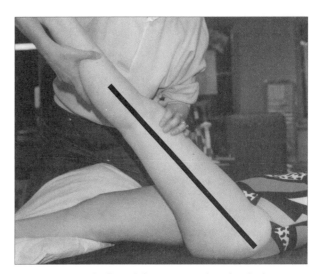

Figure 142. Passive hip flexion before treatment with Myofascial Release.

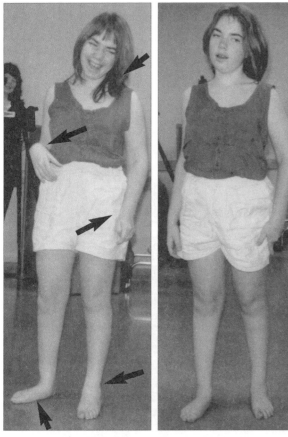

Figure 140. Before treatment with Myofascial Release; arrows point to areas of significant postural deviations.

Figure 141. After treatment with Myofascial Release.

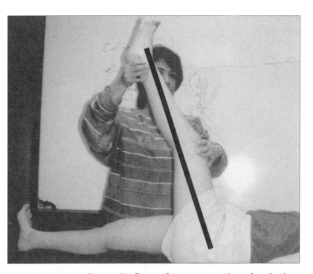

Figure 143. Increased passive hip flexion after treatment with Myofascial Release.

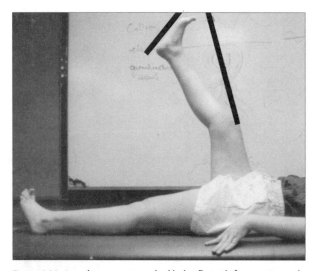

Figure 144. Active knee extension and ankle dorsiflexion before treatment with Myofascial Release.

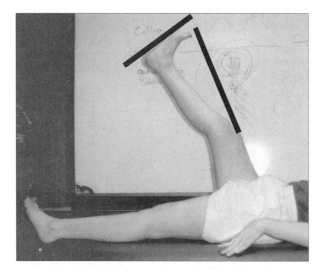

Figure 145. Increased active knee extension and ankle dorsiflexion after treatment with Myofascial Release.

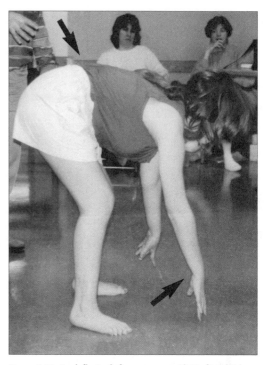

Figure 146. Trunk flexion before treatment with Myofascial Release.

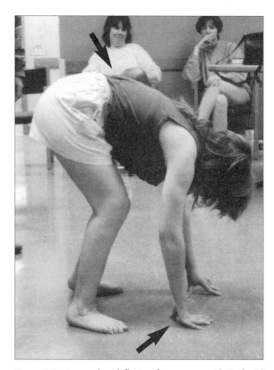

Figure 147. Increased trunk flexion after treatment with Myofascial Release.

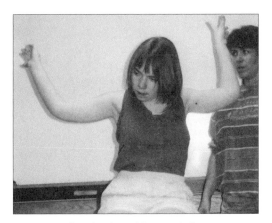

Figure 148. Bilateral total arm abduction with elbow extension before treatment with Myofascial Release. (Note that patient is not able to attain elbow extension or full shoulder abduction.)

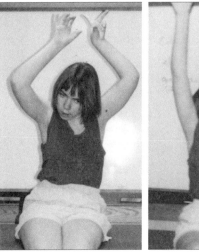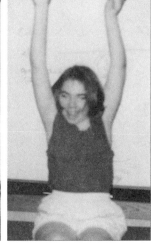

Figure 150. Bilateral shoulder elevation with elbow extension before treatment with Myofascial Release. (Note that patient is not able to attain elbow extension or full shoulder elevation.)

Figure 151. Increased bilateral shoulder elevation with increased elbow extension after treatment with Myofascial Release.

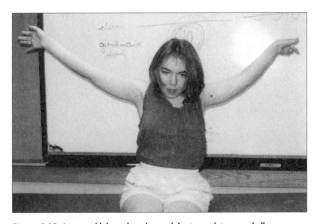

Figure 149. Increased bilateral total arm abduction with increased elbow extension after treatment with Myofascial Release.

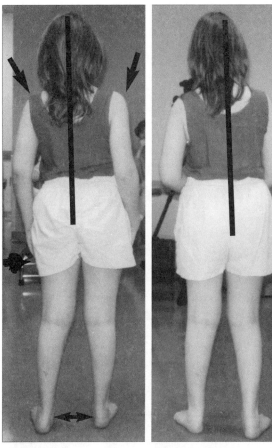

Figure 152. Midline posture before treatment with Myofascial Release.

Figure 153. Midline posture after treatment with Myofascial Release.

REFERENCES

Akeson, W.H., Amiel D., "The Connective Tissue Response to Immobility: A Study of the Chondrotin 4 and 6 Sulfate Changes in Periarticular Connective Tissue of Control and Immobilized Knees of Dogs." Clinical Orthopedics 51 (1967): 190–197

Akeson, W.H., Woo. S.L.-Y, Amiel, D., et al., "The Connective Tissue Response to Immobility: biochemical Changes in Periarticular connective Tissue of the Immobilized Rabbit Knee." Clinical Orthopedics 93 (1973): 356–362

Alexander, F.M., The Alexander Technique (New York: First Carol Publishing Group, 1989)

Aston, J., Upledger Institute, Hartford, CT 1993

Astrand, P. O., Roadhl, K., Textbook of Physiology: Physiological Bases of exercise (New York) McGrw Hill, 1977)

"Athletic Training and Sports Medicine," American Academy of Orthopedic Surgeons

Baker, W.C., Thomas, T.G., Kirkaldy-Willis, W.H., "Changes in the Articular Cartilage of the Posterior Intervertebral Joints After Anterior Fusion." Journal of Bone and Joint Surg. 51(B) (1968): 736–747

Barral, J.P., and Mercier, P., Visceral Manipulation (Seattle: Eastland Press, 1988)

Barral, J.P., the Thorax (Seattle: Eastland Press, 1991)

Barral, J.P., Urogenital Manipulation (Seattle: Eastland Press, 1993)

Barral, J.P., Visceral Manipulation II (Seattle: Eastland Press, 1999)

Berquist, R., Shaw, S., "Advanced Therapeutics," Springfield College, Springfield, MA 1978

Boone, E., "Origin and Development of the Fascial Structure," Upledger Institutes' Europe's Fourth Bi-annual Congress, University of Utrecht, Amsterdam, Holland, 1996

Bourdillion, J., Spinal Manipulation (Norwalk, CT: Appleton and Lange, 1970).

Breig, A., Biomechanics of the Central Nervous System: Some Basic Pathological Phenomena. (Chicago, IL: Yearbook Publishing Co., 1960)

Butler, D., Mobilization of the Nervous System (Melbourne: Churchill Livingstone, 1991)

Calliet, R., Soft Tissue Pain and Disability (Philadelphia: F.A. Davis, 1988)

Cantu, R., and Grodin, A., Myofasical Manipulation: Theory and Clinical Application (Gaitherburg: Aspen Publishers, 1992)

Cappelaro R., "Zero Balance I & II," Hartford, CT 1983, 1984

Castel, C., "An Introduction to the Neuroprobe: Acupuncture and TENS," Quinnipiac College, Hamden, CT 1980.

Clemente, c., A Regional Atlas of the Human Body (Baltimore, MD: Urban and Schwarzenberg, 1987)

Colton, H., Touch Therapy (New York: Kensington Publishing Co., 1983)

Cyriax, J., Textbook of Orthopedic Medicine, Vols. I & II (London: Balliere & Lindall, 1947/1977).

Dahners, L.E., "Liagament Contraction—A Correlation with Cellularity and Actin Staining" Trans. Orthop. Res. Soc. 11 (1986): 56

DeLaporte, C., Siegfried, J., " Lumbosacral Spinal Fibrosis—Spinal Arachnoidits: Its Treatment by Spinal Cord Stimulation." Spine 8 (6), (1983): 593–603

Donatelli, R., Owens-Burkhardt, W., "Effects on Immobilization on Extensibility of Periarticular Connective Tissue. Journal of Orthopedics and Sports Physical Therapy 3, 1981:67–72

Ekholm, Norback, Acta Anatomica, Basel Suppl. 15 (1951)

Enneking, W., Horowtiz, M., "The Inter-Articular Effects of Immobilization of the Human Knee," Journal of Bone and Joint Surg. 14 (5) (1972): 198–212

Enwemeka, C., "Connective Tissue Plasticity: Ultrastructural, Biomechanical and Morph metric. Effects of physical factors on intact and regenerating tendons; J. Orthopedic and Sports Physical Therapy 14(5) (Nov, 1991): 198–212

Evans, E., Eggers, G., et al., "Experimental Immobilization and Mobilization of Rat Knee Joints." Journal of Bone and Joint Surg. 42 (A) (1960): 737–758

Feldenkrais, M., Awareness Through Movement (San Francisco: Harper Collins, 1972)

Fidone, S., Eyzaguirre, C., Physiology of the Nervous System (Chicago: Yearbook Medical Publishers, 1975)

Fitton-Jackson, S., "Antecedent Phases of Matrix Formation," Structure and Function of Connective and Skeletal Tissue, 1965

Frankel, V.H., Nordin, M., Basic Biomechanics of the Musculoskeletal System (Philadelphia: Lea & Febiger, 1980)

Gamble, J.G., Edwards, D.R., Max, S.R., "Enzymatic Adaptation in Ligaments Suring Immobilization." American Journal of Sports Medicine 12 (1984): 221–228

Gray, H., Gray's Anatomy (New York: Grammercy Books of Random house, Crown Publishers, 1977)

Greenlaw, T., Ross., R., "The Development of the Rat Flexor Digital Tendon: A fine Structural Study," J. Ultrastructive Res. 18 (1967): 354–376

Gribbin, J., In Search of Schrodingers Cat: Quantum Physics and Reality (Bantam New Age, 1984)

Grieve, C., Common Vertebral Joint Problems (Edinburgh: Churchill Livingstone, 1981)

Guyton, A.C., Textbook of Medical Physiology, 7th Ed. (Philadelphia: W.B. Saunders, 1986)

Hall, B., Bone: Fracture, Repair and Regeneration Vol. 5 (Boca Raton, FL: CRC Press, Inc. 1992)

Hall, M.C., "Cartilage Changes after Experimental Immobilization of the Knee Joint for the Young Rat." Journal of Bone and Joint Surg. 45 (a) (1963): 36–52

Hardy, M., "The Biology of Scar Formation:, Physical Therapy, 69: 22–32, 1989

Heller, J., and Hanson, J., The Client's Handbook (Mt. Shasta, CA: Heller and Hellerwork, Inc.)

Hemler, M.E., Nuang, C., Schwartz, L., "The VLA Protein Family." Journal of Biologic Chemistry Vol. 262 pp. 3300–3309, March 1987

Hoffa, A.J., Technik der Massage (Stuttgart: Ferdinand Enke, 1900)

Hollinshead, H., Rosse, C., Textbook of anatomy 4th Ed. (Philadelphia: Harper Row, 1985)

Hukins, D.W., "Tissue Components," Connective Tissue Matrix Vol. I (London: McMillan Publishing, 1984)

Ingber, Donald, "The Architecture of Life," Scientific America, January 1998, pp. 48–57.

Johnson, G., "Functional Orthopedics I & II, Institute of Physical Art, New Jersey, 1987–1988

Jones, L., "Spontaneous Release by Positioning," The. D.O. 4 (1964): 109–116.

Jones, L., Strain and Counterstrain (Colorado Springs: American Academy of Osteopathy, 1981)

Jones, L., "Strain and Counterstrain" Course Notes, Hartford, CT 1991

Juhan, Deane, Job's Body, 1987

Kain, J.B., Upledger Institute Europe, Amsterdam, Holland, 1996

Kain, J.B., Weiselfish, S., "Integrated Manual therapy Protocol for Treatment of Idiopathic Scoliosis: A New Concept" Advance (Dec. 1992)

Kain, J.B., Unpublished Doctoral Thesis, an Integrated Manual Therapy Treatment Protocol: A New Approach for Treatment of Idiopathic Scoliosis. Union Institute, Cincinnati, OH 1991

Kaltenborn, F., Manual Therapy for the Extremity joints (Oslo, Norway: Olaf Norlis Bokhandel, 1976)

Korr, I., "Proprioceptors & Somatic Dysfunction," Journal of American Osteopathic Association 75 (1975): 94–104

Korr, I., and Wright, H., "Symposium on the Functional Implications of Segmental Facilitation," American Osteopathic Assoc., 47 (1947): 191–198

Kunz, K., Kunz, B., The Complete Guide to Foot Reflexology (New York: Prentice Hall, 1982)

Kurkinen, M., Vaheri, A., Roberts, P., Stenman, S., "Sequential Appearance of Fibronectin and Collagen in Experimental Granulation Tissue: Lab Invest. 43(1) (1980): 47–51

Lanier, Anatomic Record 94 (146): 311

Leach, R.A., The Chiropractic Theories (Baltimore" William & Wilkins, 1986)

Lehto, M., Duance, V.C., Restall, D., "Collagen and Fibronectin in a Healing Skeletal Muscle Injury" Journal of Bone and Joint Surg. 67 (5) (1985): 820–828

Lowen, F., and Weiselfish, S., "Biologic Analogs, Circulation Mobilization," Upledger Institute, Hartford, Ct, 1995, 1996

Lowen, F., and Weiselfish, S., "Biologic Analogs, Neural Mobilization," Upledger Institute, Hartford, CT, 1996

Lowen, F., "Practical Integration of Visceral Manipulation," Upledger Institute, Hartford, CT 1992

Lowen, F., "Visceral Manipulation II," Upledger Institute, Hartford, CT 1991

Lowen, F., "Visceral Manipulation IA," Upledger Institute, Hartford, CT 1990

MacKenzie, J., Angina Pectoris (London: Frowde, Hooder, and Stroughton, 1923) 47.

Maigne, R., Orthopedic Medicine. A New Approach to Vertebral Manipulations (Springfield, IL: Charles C. Thomas, 1972)

Maitland, G., Peripheral Manipulation (London: Butterworth, 1970)

Maitland, G., Vertebral Manipulation (London: Butterworth, 1970)

Martini, F., Fundamentals of Anatomy and Physiology (Englewood Cliffs, NJ: Prentice Hall, 1989)

McDonough, A., "Effect of Immobilization and Exercise on Articular Cartilage: A Review of Literature." Journal of Orthopedics and Sports Physical Therapy 3(1) (1981): 2–5

Mennell, J.B., Physical Treatment by Movement, Manipulation and Massage (Boston: Little, Brown & Co., 1945)

Mennell, J. McM., "History of the Development of Medical Manipulative Concepts: Medical Terminology. The Research States of Spinal Manipulative Therapy," National Institute of Neurological and Communicative Disorders and Stroke 15 (1975)

Mennell, J. Mc.M., Joint Pain (Boston: Little Brown & Co., 1964)

Mitchell, F., Moran, P., and Pruzzo, N., an Evaluation and Treatment Manual of Osteopathic Muscle Energy (Valley Park, MO: Mitchell, Moran & Pruzzo, Assoc., 1979)

Nagelschmidt, M., Becker, D., Donninghoff, N., Engelhardt, G., "Effects of Fibronectin Therapy and Fibronection Deficiency on Wound Healing: A Study in Rats" J. Trauma, 27 (11) (1987): 1267–1271

Netter, F.H., Atlas of Human Anatomy (Summit, NJ: Ciba-Geigy Corp., 1989)

Neuberger, A., Slack, H., "The Metabolism of Collagen from Liver, Bone, Skin and Tendon in Normal Rat." Biochemistry 53 (1953): 47–52

Nimi, M., Collagen—Biochemistry, Vol. I (Boca Raton, FL: CRC Press, 1988)

Nortrup, T., "The Role of Connective Tissue in Acute and Chronic Disease." Academy of Applied Osteopathy, Atlantic City, NJ, July 12, 1952

Now, V.C., Holmes, M.H. Law, W.M. "Fluid Transport and Mechanical Properties of Articular Cartilage: A Review," Journal of Biomechanics 17 (1984): 377–394

Noyes, F.R., "Functional Properties of Knee Ligaments and Alterations Induced by Immobilization," Clinical Orthopedics, 123 (1977): 210

O'Driscoll, S.W., Kumar, A., and Salter, R.B., "The Effect of Continuous Passive Motion of the Clearance of Hem arthritis." Clinical Orthopedics 176 (1983): 336

O'Driscoll, S.W., Salter, R.B., "The Induction of Neochondrogenesis in Free Intra-Articular Periosteal Autografts Under the Influence of Continuous Passive Motion." Journal of Bone and Joint Surg. 66(A) (1984): 1248

Paris, S., "Mobilization of the Spine," Physical Therapy 59(8) (1979): 988–995

Paris, S., "Spinal Manipulation Therapy," Clinical Orthopedics 179 (1983): 55–61

Parker, F., Keefer, S.C., "Gross and Histologic Changes in the Knee Joint in Rheumatoid Arthritis." Arch Path. 20(4) (1935):507.

Perlemuter, L. Waligora, J., Cahiers D'Anatome Petit Basin I (Paris, France: Masson, 1968)

Perlemuter, L. Waligora, J., Cahiers D'Anatome Petit Basin II (Paris, France: Masson & Cie , 1975)

Perlemuter, L. Waligora, J., Cahiers D'Anatome Abdomen I (Paris, France: Masson, 1976

Perlemuter, L. Waligora, J., Cahiers D'Anatome Abdomen II (Paris, France: Masson, 1987

Peterson, B., Postural Balance and Imbalance (Newark, OH: American Academy of Osteopathy, 1983).

Pischinger, A., Matrix and Matrix Regulation—Basis for a Holistic Theory in Medicine (Brussels, Belgium: Haug International, 1990)

Proctor, D.J., Guzman, N.A., "Collagen Disease and the Biosynthesis of Collagen," Hospital Practice, Dec (1977): 61–68

Rex, L., "Cranial Direct Technique," Dialogues in Contemporary Rehabilitation, Hartford, CT, 1985

Rex, L., "Myofascial Release" Course Notes, Dialogues in Contemporary Rehabilitation, Farmington, CT, 1985

Rich, A., Crick, F.H.C., "The Molecular Structure of Collagen," Journal of Molecular Medical Publishers, 1975)

Rohen, H., Yokochi, C., Color Atlas of Anatomy (Toyko, Japan: Igaku-Shoin, 1993)

Rolf, I.P., Rolfing: The Integration of Human Structures (Rochester, VT: Healing Arts Press, 1977)

Salter, R.B., Field, P., "The Effects of Continuous Compression of Living Articular Cartilage." Journal of Bone and Joint Surg. 42(A) (1960): 31–47

Salter, R.B., Bell, R.S., Kelley, F., "The Protective Effect of Continuous Passive Motion on Living Articular Cartilage in Acute Septic Arthritis: An Experimental Investigation in the Rabbit." Clinical Orthopedics 159 (1981): 223

Schoitz, E.H., "Manipulative Treatment of the Spine from a Medical-Historical Point of View, II" Ostoepathy and Chiropractic Journal of the Norwegian Medical Association 78 (1958): 429–438.

Swann, D.A., Radin, R.L., Nazimiec, M., "Role of Hyaluronic Acid in Joint Lubrication." Ann. Rheum. Dis. 33 (174): 318

Synder, G.E., "Clinical Aspects of Fascia," Academy of Applied Osteopathy yearbook (156): 65–75

The Science and Art of Joint Manipulation Vol. I & II (London: L & D Churchill, 1949/1952

Trais, A., "Effect of Persistent Pressure on the Articular Cartilage: An Experimental Study." Journal of Bone and Joint Surg. 43(B) (1961): 376–386

Travell, J.G,, Simons, D., Myofascial Pain and Dysfunction: The Trigger Point Manual (Baltimore, MD: Williams & Wilkins, 1983)

Travell, J.G., Pain Mechanisms in Connective Tissue: connective Tissues (New York: Josiah Macy, Jr. Foundation, 1951)

Travell, J., "Trigger Point Therapy" Course Notes, APTA National Conference, Washington DC, 1980

Upledger, J., Vredevogd, J.D., Cranio Sacral Therapy (Seattle: Eastland Press, 1983)

Upledger, J., "The Facilitated Segment:, Massage Therapy Journal

Upledger, J.G., "Editorial Reply on Subjectivity and Craniosacral Therapy. J. Amer. Osteo. Assoc. 78 (Feb. 1979): 25–28

Upledger, J.E., Personal Communication RE: Energy Cysts: Braina nd Spinal Cord Institute, Palms Beach Gardens, FL 1995

Weider, K., "Tragering Workshop," Regional Physical Therapy, West Hartford, CT 1990

Weiselfish, S., and Kain, J.B., "Myofascial Release for the Orthopedic and Neurologic Patient," Sturbridge, MA, 1992

Weiselfish, S., "A Systems Approach for Treatment of TMJ Dysfunction," CT State APTA Conference, 1981

Weiselfish, S., Manual Therapy with Muscle Energy Technique (West Hartford, CT: ANA Publishing, 1994)

Weiss, Jacqueline B., "Collagens and Collagenolytic Enzymes," in Connective Tissue Matrix, (John Wiley and Sons, 1984.)

Williams, I.F, McCullagh, K.G.M. Silver, I.A., "The Distribution of Type I and III Collagen and Fibronectin in the Healing Equine Tendon: Connective Tissue Research 12 (1984): 221–227

Wittlinger, J., Wittlinger G., Introduction to Dr. Vodder's Lymph Drainage Vol I (Heidlberg: Haug Publishers, 1982

Woo, S.L.-Y, Gomez, M.A. et al., "The Biomechanics and Biochemical Changes of the MCL following Immobilization and Remobilization," Journal of Bone and Joint Surg. 69A (1987): 1200–1211

Woo, S.L.-Y., Matthews, J.V., et al., "Connective Tissue Response to Immobility. Correlative Study of Biomechanical and Biochemical Measurement of Normal and Immobilized rabbit Knees." Arthritis Rheum. 18(3) (1975): 257–266.

Zohar, D., The Quantum Self (New York: Quill/William Morrow, 1990)

INDEX

ABOUT THE AUTHORS

Sharon (Weiselfish) Giammatteo, Ph.D., P.T., I.M.T., C.

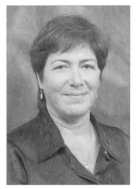

Dr. Sharon W. Giammatteo is President of CenterIMT, Center of Integrative Manual Therapy and Diagnostics, including Regional Physical Therapy in Connecticut. CenterIMT is a network of health-care clinics providing manual therapy and rehabilitation in the United States and many other countries.

Dr. W. Giammatteo earned a Ph.D. from Union Institute and University, investigating manual and cranial therapies for the neurologic client, an undergraduate degree in Advanced Health Sciences and Medicine, and a graduate degree in Clinical Neurosciences from The University of Hartford. Her Physical Therapy degree is from Wingate Institute of Physiotherapy in Israel.

Dr. W. Giammatteo is President of Dialogues in Contemporary Rehabilitation (DCR), the learning, resource, and research center for IMT in Connecticut. DCR presents over 150 seminars around the world each year. The authorized Connecticut School of Integrative Manual Therapy is located in Bloomfield, Connecticut.

Dr. W. Giammatteo developed Integrative Manual Therapy, the Integrated Systems Approach, and Integrative Diagnostics. She has taught on five continents as an expert in orthopedics, chronic pain, pediatrics, and neurologic and geriatric rehabilitation.

Jay B. Kain, Ph.D., P.T., A.T.C., I.M.T., C

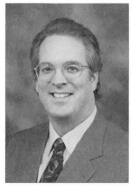

Dr. Kain is the Dean of the Connecticut School of Integrative Manual Therapy (CSIMT). He holds a Ph.D. degree from Union Institute and University in Neuromusculoskeletal Function, an M.S. degree in Biomechanics from Springfield College, and two B.S. degrees in Physical Therapy and Physical Education from Quinnipiac University and Springfield College respectively. He is also a Certified Athletic Trainer, and is the owner of Jay B. Kain Physical Therapy, Inc., located in western Massachusetts.

Dr. Kain was a ten-year cooperator for Springfield College and served on the Clinical Education Advisory Board for the Springfield College Physical Therapy Program. Additionally, Dr. Kain has been an adjunct faculty member at Russell Sage College, Troy, N.Y.

Dr. Kain teaches courses in IMT for DCR and CSIMT nationally and internationally.